"It's about time that the twenty-first-century church had some resources to enable consideration of and ministry to and with people with autism. Wherever we find ourselves—or our friends or loved ones—on the spectrum, Grant Macaskill brings his well-honed skills as a biblical scholar to bear on the realities that many in the church live with and face."
　　　　　—**Amos Yong**, *Dean of the School of Theology and the School of Intercultural Studies, Director of the Center for Missiological Research, and Professor of Theology & Mission, Fuller Theological Seminary*

"*Autism and the Church* is a thorough, humane, and quite fascinating exploration of autism which not only breaks new intellectual ground but also offers fresh possibilities for faithful practices that understand and respect the complexities of living well with autism."
　　　　　—**John Swinton**, *Chair in Divinity and Religious Studies, School of Divinity, History, and Philosophy, University of Aberdeen*

"Scientifically informed, pastorally sensitive, theologically engaged, and accessibly written, Grant Macaskill's book will greatly help Christians to 'think biblically' about the important issue of autism and about how best to enable people with autism fully to participate in the life of the church."
　　　　　—**David G. Horrell**, *Professor of New Testament Studies and Director of the Centre for Biblical Studies, University of Exeter*

"*Autism and the Church* is a well-researched and beautifully written theological reflection on a much misunderstood condition, the persons who have it, and the body of Christ to which they belong. Grant Macaskill has given the church and the world a great gift."
　　　　　—**Michael Martin**, *Associate Professor of New Testament, Lubbock Christian University*

AUTISM AND THE CHURCH
Bible, Theology, and Community

Grant Macaskill

BAYLOR UNIVERSITY PRESS

Unless otherwise stated, Scripture quotations are from the New
Revised Standard Version Bible, copyright 1989, Division of
Christian Education of the National Council of the Churches of
Christ in the United States of America. Used by permission.
All rights reserved.

Cover and book design by Savanah N. Landerholm
Cover image: Sean Brushingham, *Blue Dream*

First issued in paperback in January 2021 under ISBN
978-1-4813-1125-0

The Library of Congress has cataloged the hardcover as follows:

Library of Congress Cataloging-in-Publication Data

Names: Macaskill, Grant, author.
Title: Autism and the church : Bible, theology, and community /
  Grant Macaskill.
Description: Waco : Baylor University Press, 2019. | Includes
  bibliographical references. | Summary: "Models a Christian
  hermeneutic and practice that accommodates and cares for those
  with autism within the life of the church"-- Provided by publisher.
Identifiers: LCCN 2019015098 (print) | LCCN 2019980761 (ebook)
  | ISBN 9781481311243 (hardcover) | ISBN 9781481311267 (epub)
  | ISBN 9781481311274 (mobi) | ISBN 9781481311281 (pdf)
Subjects: LCSH: Autism--Religious aspects--Christianity. | Autism.
  Classification: LCC RC553.A88 M3188 2019 (print) |
  LCC RC553.A88 (ebook) | DDC 616.85/88200882--dc23
LC record available at https://lccn.loc.gov/2019015098
LC ebook record available at https://lccn.loc.gov/2019980761

AUTISM AND THE CHURCH
Bible, Theology, and Community

Grant Macaskill

BAYLOR UNIVERSITY PRESS

Cover and book design by Savanah N. Landerholm
Cover image: Sean Brushingham, *Blue Dream*

First issued in paperback in January 2021 under ISBN
978-1-4813-1125-0

The Library of Congress has cataloged the hardcover as follows:

Library of Congress Cataloging-in-Publication Data

Names: Macaskill, Grant, author.
Title: Autism and the church : Bible, theology, and community /
  Grant Macaskill.
Description: Waco : Baylor University Press, 2019. | Includes
  bibliographical references. | Summary: "Models a Christian
  hermeneutic and practice that accommodates and cares for those
  with autism within the life of the church"-- Provided by publisher.
Identifiers: LCCN 2019015098 (print) | LCCN 2019980761 (ebook)
  | ISBN 9781481311243 (hardcover) | ISBN 9781481311267 (epub)
  | ISBN 9781481311274 (mobi) | ISBN 9781481311281 (pdf)
Subjects: LCSH: Autism--Religious aspects--Christianity. | Autism.
  Classification: LCC RC553.A88 M3188 2019 (print) |
  LCC RC553.A88 (ebook) | DDC 616.85/88200882--dc23
LC record available at https://lccn.loc.gov/2019015098
LC ebook record available at https://lccn.loc.gov/2019980761

For Kenny, Anna, Bella, Archie, and Hettie Robertson

CONTENTS

✻

ACKNOWLEDGMENTS

This book could not have been written without the extraordinary generosity and patience of a host of people. Carey Newman and others at Baylor University Press have been supportive of my research into autism from the beginning and have gone several extra miles to bring it through the publishing process as smoothly as possible. By the time you read this, their patience and generosity will have been stretched to their limit and my gratitude will be even greater than it is now. I could not have written the book without the input of colleagues at the University of Aberdeen—especially John Swinton, Brian Brock, and Léon van Ommen, all of whom work on the theological evaluation of autism. While these colleagues have been directly influential on the work, other colleagues have contributed in all sorts of ways to my reflection on the issues and have, of course, been wonderful academic friends: Tom Greggs, Phil

Ziegler, Paul Nimmo, Katy Hockey, Jutta Leonhardt-Balzer, Don Wood, Joachim Schaper, Tomas Bokedal, Daniel Jackson, Ken Jeffrey, Katie Cross, and Sir Iain Torrance. Within the wider environment of the University of Aberdeen, George Coghill, Paula Sweeney, Andrew Dilley, Michael Brown, Pete Stollery, Clare Davidson, and our amazing chaplains, Marylee Anderson and David Hutchison, have all been more important than they probably know. There is simply not space to list all of those outside of Aberdeen who have contributed to the development of the book, but I will mention Micheal O'Siadhail, Ivor Davidson, David Horrell, Mike Bird, Jamie Davies, Kirstyn Oliver, Joanne Leidenhag, Sarah Douglas, Mark Stirling, Jared Michelson, Dave Redfern, Alasdair I. and Cathie Macleod, Kenny and Anna Robertson, and all involved in the Additional Needs Alliance. As always, Pete and Jo Nixon (and Finlay and Toby) and Kenny and Anna MacLeod deserve thanks for their continuing support and friendship. My wider family has also continued to be supportive, both my parents and my brothers, Roddy and Scott.

Above all, I thank my wife, Jane, without whose patience and support I could not do this work.

INTRODUCTION
Autism and Church

In the past, one heard almost nothing of autism. The condition only began to be labeled and studied in the early twentieth century, but even then, it was considered extremely rare, affecting perhaps 1 in 10,000 persons. In recent years, however, the estimated incidence has risen dramatically, to the point where the condition is believed to affect anything from 1 in 200 to 1 in 50 persons. The reasons for this increase will be considered in the course of this book — they are less sinister than is sometimes alleged — but the figures bear out what many readers will recognize: autism is common, even if the actual diagnosis rates are still catching up with its estimated incidence. It is so common, in fact, that almost every Christian community will experience its effects in some way, whether through members who are autistic or have autistic children or through interaction with the wider society within which the church is located. That is why a book like this is necessary.

Most Christians consider the Bible to be the word of God and to be normative for their thought and life. What they mean by the expression "word of God" may vary between different traditions, and these differences have a significant bearing on how the Bible's normative role is conceived, but most Christians will consider the Bible to play a decisive role in how they think about the issues they encounter. They will want to know what it means to "think biblically" about these issues. But how does one think biblically about something like autism, when the condition itself was not known as such in the ancient world? The biblical writers had no category that matched the modern definition of autism, which means that we cannot find texts or passages that obviously inform our thinking about it. Given this, should we try to find ways in which the phenomena of autism might be visible in the text, just labeled (and perhaps identified) differently? Some have tried to do exactly this, either suggesting that certain biblical characters were obviously "on the spectrum" (I will explain that term in chapter 1) or, quite differently, that what we label as autism is actually symptomatically equivalent to demon possession. These attempts may be well intended, but they are highly problematic, as we will see in the course of this book. I will suggest, instead, that we have to listen more carefully to the biblical material to identify principles that might shape our evaluation of autism and also our interactions with those who experience the condition (or, for those who are themselves autistic, their experience of interactions with "neurotypicals").[1] As we will see, this is not just about the content of particular biblical passages, although there will be a fair amount of close engagement with these, but also about our underlying ways of thinking about what we are doing as interpreters of the Bible, and how our interpretations can be mapped onto our lives today. The principles and observations that will be discussed along the way are not all unique to the study of autism; in many cases, they bear more broadly on how Christians think about developments in the modern world, particularly the world of medicine and health care.

This book is a work of research. It involves the exploration of issues that have not been considered in such depth before and, in many ways, represents the pursuit of an entirely new field of inquiry.[2] In writing it, though, I am conscious of its immediate relevance to a range of readerships, and I have sought to write in such a way that it will be accessible to as many of these as possible. Often, as researchers, we write for other members of the research community; we generate highly technical literature that takes the field forward in important but incremental ways. Such literature is largely unintelligible to those who have not been trained in certain technical skills or schooled in certain discussions. Sometimes this research will be brokered to a wider audience by those who occupy mediating roles between the academic and nonacademic communities. In medical research, for example, clinicians and support workers will often bear the responsibility of sharing current research with patients and families, sometimes by generating further literature that is more widely accessible. In the case of theology and biblical scholarship, that mediating role is more typically associated with pastors and Christian leaders and the seminaries in which they may be trained. Because autism is still making its way into widespread public awareness, however, there may be nothing in place to broker research into autism systematically within the churches. Some individuals and families may find themselves in church communities that deal well with the condition, but others may feel that they are dealing with it alone; clinicians and healthcare providers may be aware of the distinctive needs that mark Christian patients, but they may have no idea how to meet those needs. In writing this book, I am deeply conscious of the need to minimize the barriers between such individuals and the research itself, without sacrificing necessary technical depth.

This has affected the way I present the material. All biblical scholarship, including that oriented toward practical theological discussion, must deal at points with technical matters of language—nuances of Greek, Hebrew, and occasionally Aramaic, at both lexical and syntactical levels—but these can be explained for the nonspecialist. The barriers to understanding can be minimized by transliterating the characters of those languages into the Latin alphabet, so that readers can at least know what the technical material under discussion sounds like. Where I interact with matters of language, this is exactly what I do, and with more explanation of grammar than would be necessary if I were writing for other New Testament scholars. This decision reflects my awareness that even academic readers of this book will not necessarily be specialists in the biblical languages or the methodologies of exegesis, the practices by which we analyze the text. Similarly, all scholarship must today interact with a vast amount of secondary literature on our primary texts; any given part of the Bible will have been the subject of hundreds, or even thousands, of books and articles. Some interaction with this will be necessary to satisfy the demands of stringent research, but it is unlikely to be helpful for many readers and may, in fact, obscure the matters of real importance. Such discussion will be located, then, in endnotes and will be carefully limited to ensure that what is included is only what is genuinely necessary.

In the opening chapter, I will survey historical and recent research into autism, in order to ensure that readers are aware of (1) how autism is presently understood within the scientific literature and (2) which accounts of autism are now considered to be problematic. There is always a danger, when condensing a massive body of literature into a summary of sorts, that specialists in particular areas will feel their research is not well represented. There is also a danger that those who are themselves autistic will feel that their distinctive experiences of the condition are not appropriately represented. This is probably unavoidable, but I hope that the chapter will provide a helpful entry point into the literature on autism, including the literature emerging from within the autism community, rather than serving as a definitive account for any serious reader. Even within the context of this book, it will not be the only discussion of the characteristics of autism, some details of which will be woven into later chapters. As part of this chapter, though, I will offer some general reflections on how autism may bear on the experience of people in churches.

In chapter 2, I will propose a set of principles that should govern how the Bible is read in relation to autism. I will contrast these principles with problematic approaches to applying the Bible to autism, including those that identify autism with the demonic and those that suggest a Christian response to autism should involve the expectation of healing.

In chapter 3, I will build on these principles, arguing that the gospel challenges the values by which we naturally ascribe worth and honor to socially impressive persons. This obligates us to reconsider the importance of those with autism in the church, who are typically marginalized, undervalued, or treated with contempt. I will also note, however, that the sinful ways in which we intuitively value strength and social capital remain stubbornly present within the church, which is not an automatically safe place for people who are different (such as those with autism).

In chapter 4, I will build further upon these observations by considering how a church that values its members, including those with autism, should accommodate the particular social and sensory challenges its members might have. This will involve some recognition of how the language of weakness is applied by

Paul to the obligation of Christians to use their freedom in ways that avoid harming the sensitivities of others.

In chapter 5, I will discuss the difficult topic of the problems that can co-occur with autism for many individuals, notably anxiety, depression, and addiction. I will seek to contextualize these within the presentation of the gospel in the New Testament and will devote considerable space to discussing how the themes of "weakness" and "flesh" are used within the redemptive accounts of the New Testament, notably Paul's.

In chapter 6, I will discuss four smaller topics that have repeatedly surfaced in my research into autism and that need to be dealt with, even briefly. These are: the question of how parents of profoundly autistic persons think about the limits on their children's ability to profess or confess faith, the question of how those who find prayer to be difficult might make use of biblical resources such as the psalms, the question of how autism and gender identity relate, and the question of whether persons with autism might read the Bible differently than others.

In the conclusion, I will offer some final reflections, intended to pull together some of the strands of the book and to highlight some of the themes that have surfaced in different ways in different chapters.

This is avowedly not a definitive or final study of autism and Christian community, considered in biblical and theological terms. It is an attempt to consider the issues in some depth, in a somewhat exploratory fashion, written in full awareness that some of my suggestions may be wrong or open to challenge, while others do not go far enough. There are issues that I hope to consider in greater depth in a later study, particularly around the question of language use, and these have been previewed here but hardly analyzed in full. I am also deeply conscious that this work contributes to a conversation that has barely started and that needs to begin to cross boundaries. My work needs to be part of a conversation with other disciplines in theology and with those in the churches who actually deal with autism as a pastoral or personal reality. It also needs to be part of a conversation with practitioners in medicine and in public health care, who do not necessarily understand how religious value systems bear upon the experience of those in the process of being diagnosed or supported; this may lead some practitioners to avoid involvement in those processes. In due course, this work also needs to be part of a conversation that takes place across religious boundaries: we need to reflect on how these issues play out in other religious contexts (some of which share some scriptural resources with Christianity) and how the different religious traditions might learn from each other. This book will, I hope, be an important step in furthering the conversation, but that is all it is—a step.

I am conscious in writing this book that some readers will feel that their own ways of thinking about autism are being challenged and, perhaps, dismissed. This may be as true of the medical practitioner as it is of the pastor, for while I generally assume the validity of the clinical research into autism as the starting point for my own work, I will also challenge some of the language that is frequently used in that research. All I can ask is that readers give the material a fair hearing and be "critically open-minded" to my claims.

I hope this will also be true of readers with autism and their families. Those with autism are often justifiably concerned about the way the condition is described in research literature or represented by well-intentioned advocates who, nevertheless, lack firsthand experience of the condition. When, for example, autistic people are described as "lacking empathy" or as incapable of understanding "nonliteral" use of language, they feel misrepresented or wrongly labeled. They are made to feel "other."[3] Often, autistic persons feel that such labels are just further examples of neurotypicals imposing their categories on those who differ from them. The problem is compounded by the diversity with which autism is experienced: descriptions are often either overly general or overly specific, in ways that simply do not describe a particular person's experience of autism. For my part, I can only ask that autistic readers will trust that this book has not been written out of purely academic interest, but out of personal experience and investment. I do not think it would be appropriate, at this point, to discuss my experience of autism in detail, because the experience is not mine alone and those who have shared it with me should not have to be pulled into this book. I recognize, though, that it is a particular experience of autism, involving what would widely be identified as "Asperger syndrome." This is a very different experience of autism in comparison to the experiences of others, such as my colleague Brian Brock, whose son is profoundly autistic.[4] I have been sensitive throughout the writing of this book to the danger of discussing autism only in terms that correspond to my own experience, and I have sought to keep other experiences in view. I leave it to readers to decide whether I have done so successfully, but I hope their judgment will be shaped by an awareness that this study emerges from personal experience, both good and bad.

This spectrum of experiences also bears on the way in which I speak about faith in this book. At some points I will speak of "believers," and at other points I will speak of the families and caregivers[5] of persons with profound autism. I am committed to the importance of "faith" within Christianity and to the experience of salvation, but I am also aware that many who are themselves believers care for autistic persons who are minimally verbal, whose cognitive awareness of the substance of Christian faith is, at this point, beyond our capacity to investigate. I discuss this in chapter 6, in some depth, but throughout the writing of the book I have been aware of the fact that I am dealing with a range of experiences that map differently onto the experience of Christian belief. It is impossible to do justice to this at every point, and so I would ask readers to be generous and patient throughout the study, allowing that some parts speak immediately to the experiences of believers with autism, and others to how the community should treat the autistic family members of believers.

Finally, there is a widespread and understandable sensitivity to the need for "person-centered" language to be used in all talk about autism. Rather than speaking about "autistic" individuals, many (especially those who work in health care) prefer to speak about "persons with autism," in order to avoid diminishing the importance or reality of the personhood associated with those who experience the condition. Those who have seen the recent television series *Atypical* (which is far from perfect as a representation of autism but still contains some valuable insights) may remember a conversation involving the father of a teenager with autism and others in the parent support group, in which the father is castigated for transgressing this principle.[6] In the context of the show, it is a window into the experience of a father who loves his son but who struggles to stay on top of the challenges that accompany the situation. For us, it is an interesting representation of the problems that arise from all attempts to talk or write sensitively about autism. Sometimes the language of "persons with autism" feels stiff or forced and can even intensify the sense that autism is being categorized as something "other." A recent study conducted in the UK found that many who are themselves autistic dislike this particular term, since it suggests that their autism is detachable from their personhood; instead, they consider their personhood and identity to be distinctively and inescapably shaped by their autism.[7] For them, the adjective "autistic," sometimes used as a stand-alone substantive, is the most affirming and appropriate term with which to be identified. The study concluded that "no single way of describing autism" is universally accepted and that the disagreements over usage are "deeply entrenched."[8] These disagreements reflect the tensions that are often felt between the healthcare and research communities and those who are themselves autistic. It will be very clear in what follows that I am gravely concerned by the ways in which the personhood of those with autism is often unwittingly minimized by the descriptions of the condition. I hope that this will contextualize any points where I choose to use the term "autistic" rather than a lengthier alternative. My own use of language will reflect the diversity recognized in the study noted above: sometimes I will use the expression preferred by healthcare professionals ("persons with autism"), but often I will use the terminology preferred by those who would label themselves "actually autistic."[9]

1

✳

REAL AUTISM
Characteristics and Explanations

Autism is a lifelong, developmental disability that affects how
a person communicates with and relates to other people, and
how they experience the world around them.[1]

The core definition given above is taken directly from the
home page of the UK National Autistic Society. Despite
some differences in the clinical and diagnostic literature used in
North America and the rest of the world,[2] it is one that would be
endorsed by healthcare practitioners around the world. While
there is some debate about the use of the word "disability,"
which will be considered later in this chapter, the definition provides a useful starting point for thinking about what the term
"autism" labels. Some elements of the statement may be familiar
to readers, particularly the identification of social and communicative differences in those affected by the condition, but other
elements may be surprising. Few people are aware that autism

involves complex and varied sensory issues that affect how the person experiences and even perceives the world. Smells, sights, sounds, colors—all of these can be quite different for the person with autism, perhaps because their sensory information is differently "filtered" than it is for other people. Increasingly, in fact, this is seen as a (or even *the*) key element for how we understand the condition, rather than a side effect, which is how it was treated in some earlier research.

The word "autism" itself can be traced back to some of the earliest research into the condition, which was carried out in the period after the First World War and continued into the second.[3] The word was brought into German, and then into English, from the Greek word *autos*, which means "self/himself/herself/itself," depending on the case and context of its usage. The term "autistic" was applied to children who appeared to be compromised in their social and interactive abilities; a person who was "autistic" appeared to be shut off from the world, self-focused or even self-contained, compromised in their ability to interact with the "other." When understood in this original or etymological sense, the word is highly problematic as a label, but it is unlikely to be changed, and, in any case, few people use the word with an awareness of its etymology. For most, "autism" is simply the word that labels this particular condition.

The identification of autism as a "lifelong, developmental" condition is vital to our perception of its causes and to the prospects for those who experience it. The most reliable current research indicates that autism is the result of the expression of genes,[4] even if other factors may be involved in this expression. It is not a disease triggered by the exposure of infants to certain toxins,[5] or a psychological disorder caused by parenting dynamics,[6] but a genetically linked neurological condition, which involves a demonstrably different neural development than that seen in the wider population. Autism will not "go away" with the right treatment, although most people with autism can adapt, learning skills that allow them to navigate and understand social expectations that are intuitive to others, and to learn how to manage the relentless flood of sensory data that others filter out.

Some readers, whether because they have been persuaded by the claims that autism is a result of immunization programs or because they are committed to the possibility of divine healing (or even deliverance), may already be bristling at the assertion that it is a lifelong developmental condition. These particular issues will be considered in more depth later in the book. Here I will simply note two things and ask that readers reflect carefully upon them before deciding that that this book is hopelessly entangled with establishment-sponsored research. First, the evidence that autism is a developmental condition associated with differences in the physical neurology of the person is strong: there are demonstrable physical differences between those with autism and the wider population.[7] While the model of the brain as a computer is really quite deficient,[8] it is still helpful to consider autism as a condition in which the neural "wiring" is different from the wider population. Second, while these differences are demonstrable through clinical investigation, they are not *obviously* visible. People with autism do not look physically any different than other people. This is important, because it means that we will (perhaps subconsciously) assume that the person has developed "normally" and that any differences in behavior or experience are superficial and can be treated or undone. To illustrate this point, let me use an example from my own wider family. I have a relative with Down syndrome, whose sister has autism (of a kind that would commonly be referred to as Asperger syndrome). Because my relative with Down syndrome presents the usual physical characteristics that accompany that condition, few people would expect that her condition could be healed. Healing would change her entire appearance and, of course, her personality (which no one would want to see altered, because she is quite delightful). It is *obvious* that she has a developmental condition. By contrast, it is not *physically* obvious that her sister is a person with autism. It is easier to believe that she could be healed, or that her condition arose at some point during childhood, because there is nothing on the surface of her anatomy to indicate that her condition can be traced all the way back to the expression of her genes, even though this is the most likely explanation for her autism.[9]

Autism as a Spectrum

One of the most important developments in autism research has been the shift from using the term as a label for a very specific condition, marked by particular and quite severe symptoms, to using it for a spectrum of conditions, with symptoms varying in kind and severity. "Classical autism," in which persons would be profoundly compromised in their social and communicative development, is now seen to be one particular point on a much wider spectrum, in which a range of characteristics may present themselves, and to varying degrees.

The move toward seeing autism as a spectrum of conditions is *the* key factor in the dramatic rise of the estimated incidence of the condition. When the label "autism" was associated only with a particular and quite severe point on the spectrum, the estimated incidence was understandably low: 1 in 10,000. Once researchers began to use the term for a wider range of conditions that had certain similarities to classical autism but were usually less severe in their effects, the estimated incidence naturally rose. In the English-speaking world, that shift really began in the 1980s, but took decades to filter down into frontline clinical activity and then into popular awareness. As this process has moved forward, the estimated incidence has grown dramatically, to the point where it is now common to hear figures like 1 in 200 or even 1 in 50. Importantly, these are only estimates: the actual diagnosis figures are still catching up, as many are only now coming forward for an adult diagnosis (since the condition was not known when they were growing up) and the diagnosis services are creaking under the weight of demand. In many areas in the United Kingdom, for example, the waiting time for diagnosis, from referral to consultation, can stretch to several years. This is an important issue for pastors and churches to be aware of: there may be persons in any congregation who are as yet undiagnosed. This requires distinct pastoral care, one strand of which must be to recognize that proper diagnosis requires proper diagnostic expertise. It is dangerously easy for pastors and church communities to diagnose one of their members as being "on the spectrum," a judgment that usually goes with denigrating the person's value or dismissing them as "eccentric." Sometimes a professional diagnosis is not practical; even the UK's National Autistic Society recognizes that self-diagnosis may be important for those who do not decide to enter a formal diagnosis process or who are on the lengthy waiting list.[10] But this means diagnosis by the people themselves, not by their church or pastor.

The shift toward speaking of an autism spectrum (older literature tended to use "autistic spectrum") was associated particularly with the work of Lorna Wing,[11] whose categories were informed by the pioneering work of Hans Asperger.[12] Asperger's work was broadly contemporary with that of Leo Kanner, whose research dominated the perception of autism for decades. Kanner focused on those with the profound condition—the 1 in 10,000 who were once identified exclusively as "autistic"—and proposed various explanations for the condition that were "psychogenic" in character: autism, in other words, was a disorder that arose through social and psychological influence, notably that of the mother. Classical autism is still sometimes referred to as Kanner's syndrome, because of his role in researching the condition. Hans Asperger, by contrast, worked with less profoundly affected children, whose positive qualities he was careful to document. Asperger's early research took place at a time when Germany was moving toward the political environment associated with the Third Reich. Accounts of Asperger's work have typically represented him as acting to protect vulnerable children from the policies of the Reich, but evidence has emerged more recently that calls this into question, suggesting that he collaborated with the Nazis.[13] For those who have viewed Asperger as the champion of a more positive approach to autism, this has proved troubling. Whatever the truth of this might be, Kanner's work was widely influential for decades, while Asperger's went largely unknown in the English-speaking world until Wing's research began to draw upon and publicize its categories. It is for this reason that the term Asperger syndrome (or disorder) began to be used of those who presented some similar characteristics to those with profound classical autism but who appeared not to be as significantly affected. Such persons might previously have been labeled as eccentric or difficult, but were not reliant on lifelong care, as those with profound autism were.

While Wing's work was crucial in establishing the concept of the autism spectrum in Anglophone medical practice, Temple Grandin's writings were arguably more influential in publicizing the concept. Grandin, herself autistic, is a brilliant researcher into animal welfare and husbandry (particularly housing environments), but her writings on autism helped to make the concept of the spectrum known within the wider population. She gave the public a first-person account of how her brain worked and opened the way for a more constructive conversation about autism and the spectrum of traits with which it presents itself.

The term "spectrum" needs some further comment before we consider the various characteristics that it tends to present. It runs the risk of being understood in linear and one-dimensional terms, like a progressive shading from white to black, through gray. This assumption of linearity is compounded by the fact that the word is often used in conjunction with some value-laden qualifiers, such as "high-functioning" and "low-functioning." This can lead us to think that the spectrum is simply a range of progressively more severe characteristics, consistent in character but not in extremity, and always directly mapped onto the functioning of the person as a whole, which is basically subject to grading categories such as "high" and "low" (which, in turn, often lead to a judgment on the worth of a person). In truth, the term "spectrum" really labels the diversity of both the symptoms that might be associated with autism and their severity. Properly, its value lies more in its rejection of a concept of autism that is too narrow and singular than in its inference of linearity or its grading of severity. In fact, the language of "high-" and "low-functioning" will itself have to be interrogated theologically, something we will do later in this book. Whatever we might make of such language, though, it is always particular to the various characteristics present in the individual. One person might be labeled as "high-functioning" because they have been able to pursue a successful career, even though some of their autistic characteristics might entirely impair their ability to do certain activities or to deal with certain situations. They may lose the ability to speak because of sensory overload if someone nearby is wearing perfume or is whistling. Their relationship with a spouse may sometimes be difficult because they do not intuitively perceive certain expectations or reciprocate certain needs. In certain situations, they may struggle to function well, while in others they may excel. It is certainly the case that some autistic people, due to the nature and extent of their characteristics, will always be dependent on caregivers, but it may not be helpful to think of this in terms of "low function," since doing so means making a number of judgments on what constitutes "proper" function. As far as possible, the language of "high function" and "low function" will be avoided in this book because it is so laden with these kinds of judgments.

Characteristics of the Autism Spectrum

What, then, are the characteristics of the autism spectrum, and why might they be seen as connected, rather than as distinct conditions? It would be possible to itemize a list of such characteristics and say that the presence of several of them is indicative, if not actually diagnostic, of an autism spectrum disorder. This is part of the guidance that is given for the identification of autism.[14] For present purposes, however, it will probably be more helpful to cluster the characteristics to help illustrate the connections between them. It will, I hope, become clear fairly quickly that the various characteristics may be wrapped up with each other.

The best-known (rather than "most obvious") cluster of characteristics of the autism spectrum relates to social interaction and communication. Autistic people typically do not perceive certain forms of nonverbal communication in the same way that others do, and, probably because of this, their capacity to participate intuitively in social interaction can be affected. They can range from the person who appears to be socially awkward or to miss certain cues through to the profoundly affected person, who seems to be almost shut off from the world. There are certain behavioral tendencies that go with this. Persons with autism often find eye contact difficult, or their eye contact is unusual and seen by others as "unnatural": they may hold eye contact for longer than is usually considered appropriate, or may focus on another part of the face (such as the mouth), or may only occasionally look at the eyes of the other person. They may not perceive an emotional or affective state to be present in another person because they do not pick up on the body language or facial expressions that accompany such emotions; consequently, they may not respond intuitively to someone's need for comfort or congratulations. Participation in social customs will often also be difficult. Greeting, for example, typically involves eye contact, facial expressions, and some kind of physical contact such as an embrace or a handshake; these things generate a sense of bond between individuals. For those with autism, however, such practices may not be intuitively meaningful or may even be quite uncomfortable. In some cases, the attempt to force eye contact onto a person with autism can be seriously distressing; there are countless horror stories of teachers or therapists seeking to do exactly this with a child who may not yet have been diagnosed, and even some stories of this being a deliberate treatment strategy.[15] It is also something that can be difficult for an adult attending a church and being greeted at the door.

The second cluster of characteristics concerns the use of language by those with autism. Both language acquisition and language use tend to be different for those with autism. Again, this presents in a range of ways and to varying degrees of severity. In profound cases, those with autism can be effectively nonverbal and can remain so for their whole lives; this usually goes with a need for lifelong care. In less extreme cases, the use of language can be quite precise, often avoiding (or misinterpreting) figures of speech that are layered with meaning beyond the proper plain sense of the words used. This is often described as an "overly literal" use of language, but that is a rather imprecise label, since it really describes the perceived referentiality between the words used and what they are used of.[16] Actually, persons with autism may have no difficulty in understanding or recognizing metaphor, which is not a literal form of speech. What they often have difficulty with are embedded idioms, especially ones that reflect affective or emotional matters, or uses of speech that run contrary to the plain sense of the words, such as irony or sarcasm. These uses of speech are better labeled as "imprecise" or "unsystematic": they violate the natural principles of the language in use. They are something that people use all the time, of course: they are part and parcel of creative communication, and it is an element in most social interaction to break the normal practices of language with irony, sarcasm, punning, and so on. Such uses of language can be difficult for those with autism, however, at least until they have learned to identify the idioms or wordplays at work.

One of the things that is linked to both of the clusters just described is a tendency to use language with a degree of honesty that others find difficult. Autistic people often do not observe the social conventions by which people politely veil what they really think behind a form of words that does not exactly correspond to truth. There is, for example, no shortage of stories about partners who have asked a leading question, looking for affirmation, and have received an answer that was more honest than they had wanted.

Q. "Does this outfit make me look fat?"
A. "Yes."

This degree of honesty can be seen as a virtue, but it is not a welcome virtue when a partner needs some encouragement. Outside of those intimate relationships, when it is encountered without context or explanation, it can cause serious hostility. When, for example, a colleague shares an idea for how to develop the business, and the person with autism simply articulates the truth about why it will not work and should not be considered further, the results can be unpleasant. The colleague thinks the person with autism is rude, arrogant, and dismissive; the person with autism simply thinks they are being helpful. In a church environment, such honesty can be perceived as quite hurtful, since it may well be directed toward an expressed viewpoint or cherished practice that is held dear by a fellow Christian.

The third cluster of characteristics is associated with systems. Generally, autistic people are drawn to systems and often like to deal systematically with their interests. Some of the common stereotypes of the person with autism are connected to these traits, whether they involve an interest in mathematics or physics or an obsession with trains and timetables. This is sometimes described as a "systematizing tendency":[17] autistic persons will often seek to identify systematic elements in the world and interact with them in a way that reflects this identification. This extends to matters of personal routine and schedule: those with autism will usually prefer routines and tend to find any disruption of a routine, or of a predecided plan for the day, quite distressing. Much of this seems to be linked to an underlying need to achieve some kind of control over one's life and environment. Systems are predictable, and one can take comfort in that predictability; seeing the world in systemic terms allows at least a semblance of control over its unpredictable qualities. One particular subcategory of autism that has recently begun to be discussed ("demand-avoidant autism" or "pathological demand avoidance")[18] is generally regarded as manifesting basic anxieties about whether the person will be able to maintain control of their environment if they take on particular roles or commitments. Of course, the world cannot be entirely systematized, and those same anxieties are often commonly felt by those with autism as they deal with the overwhelmingly unpredictable world, and not least with social interactions that make no systemic sense to them. As will be discussed in chapter 5 of this book, these tendencies can be linked to the genuinely dark side of autism, as systematic interests turn to obsessions, or as anxieties brought on by the chaos of the world create a level of distress that often drives the person to substance abuse.

The last cluster of characteristics is probably the least known in the general population, but it is also probably the most important. Those with autism typically have sensory issues that affect the way they perceive and experience the world. Sometimes their sensory experience can be duller than that of the wider population, so that they need excessive sensory input; often, though, their sensory experience is dramatically more intense. Smells that are barely noticeable to another person will be overwhelming; sounds that are scarcely detectable may be deafening, or penetrating, or distressing. The touch that others would find delightful is awful to one person with autism; the attempt of a parent or lover to show affection may cause another to recoil. Certain clothes may be unwearable because of the way that they feel; certain colors may cause anxiety.

It is not simply that these sensory data seem to be louder, brighter, or stronger than they are for other people; they are actually perceived differently. Sometimes the data may be quiet, but may still be distressing and disrupt all other sensory processing. The faint whine of an electrical appliance or charger or the sound of someone eating chips may occur at a low level of volume, but it can cut through all other sensory inputs and elicit obsessional reactions within the mind. The research on this suggests that the problem is not with the senses themselves, as if the neurons in question are just more sensitive than they are in other people. Rather, the interpretive filters that allow our brains to process and prioritize the mass of sensory information that is constantly flowing into us appear not to work in the same way that they do in the wider population.[19] Instead of the brain screening out the sensory data that are not important and focusing on interpreting what has been identified as genuinely important, the brain is flooded by everything—or at least by much more of the information than it can really make sense of. In one sense, this means that those with autism might have a purer perception of the world around them than others, but a person with this purer perception might be likened to someone who has just been capsized and plunged underwater by a massive wave: the brain is simply overwhelmed by everything that is rushing into it.

This is often referred to as sensory overload, and it is simply exhausting for the person with autism. The flood of information creates a state of anxiety and distress, often resulting in "meltdowns." Meltdowns are often confused with tantrums, especially in children, but they are quite different in character, most notably in that they are not oriented toward getting something that has been withheld. Autistic persons may seek to deal with sensory overload by performing behaviors that they find comforting: this is often referred to as "stimming," and may vary from rubbing a part of the body to spinning around or flapping limbs. Their capacity to manage interactions with other people may be severely compromised at such times, and they may simply need to be left alone. It is possible that some of the apparently violent or self-destructive behavior of the profoundly autistic is itself a form of stimming, triggered by certain sensory factors.

Increasingly, research into autism sees the sensory dimension to the condition as having significant explanatory potential. The social difficulties encountered may be connected to difficulties in differentiating the importance of sensory data, or to differences in how they are processed; the interest in systems may reflect a way of imposing control onto a world that is simply overwhelming. However far this may be taken as an explanatory account, it is certainly the case that the sensory aspect of autism is no longer seen to be a quirky side-phenomenon of the condition, but as a central element, with the clinical literature and accepted definitions reflecting this.[20]

It is important to be clear that these characteristics can be present in an almost limitless variety of combinations and with varying extents of adaptation. One person may be fine with sounds but sensitive to smell or touch, while another may have the opposite difficulty. One person may struggle with certain *kinds* of sounds but have no problem with others that inflict torture on someone else. One person may have learned how to manage the sensory flood, at least when in public, while another may still be at the mercy of the inputs. The same can be said about each of the clusters. It is often said that if you have met one person with autism, you have met one person with autism. The experiences of one can seldom, if ever, be transferred to another. It is vitally important for churches and their leaders to recognize this: they must respond to the individual person and their distinctive qualities. At the same time, it is appropriate to speak of these clusters because there is a certain common-ality that can be boiled down to a paraphrase of the definition cited at the beginning of the chapter: autistic people experience difficulty participating in the social and sensory world of the neurotypical.

Is Autism a Disability?

As noted at the beginning of the chapter, autism is typically defined as a "disability." This is a somewhat sensitive point in the discussion of the condition (and readers may already have noted my own preference for the term "condition"). Many who are affected by autism embrace the condition positively and prefer to speak of neurodiversity: people have diverse kinds of neural wiring, and one kind should not be seen as normal and another as abnormal. Rather, we should affirm the diversity. Viewed in such terms, autism might be seen as difference rather than disability. Some of the differences, in fact, might be quite empowering: the neurotype of an autistic person might allow them to be highly capable of certain tasks that would be difficult for a nonautistic person (a "neurotypical"), whether because of their distinctive sensory abilities or their capacity to detect, analyze, and construct systems.

Several points of caution should be noted, however. First, these identifications may be fine for someone who would be labeled as "high-functioning,"[21] but they are less easily applied to the person with profound autism, who may require lifelong care and whose freedoms and experiences may be dramatically impaired by the condition. In fact, for the parent or caregiver of such a person, denying that they are disabled may be highly offensive and dismissive of the enormous challenges that they face every day. Second, in practical terms the identification of a disability opens a realm of medical support and care that is otherwise closed; labels are often unhelpful things, but sometimes they allow us to access help that can make a significant difference. Third, it is important not to be naïve about the compromising limitations that affect those with autism. We need to be honest about our capacity to recognize nonverbal cues or to deal appropriately with sensory experience; as we will see in the conclusion, this bears on how autistic people might function within roles of leadership or responsibility within the community of the Christian church. It must not be allowed to exclude them from such positions, but the reality of the challenges involved should not be minimized. In fact, many within the autistic community press for the recognition that neurodiversity and disability are not mutually exclusive categories. The positive significance of diversity can be affirmed alongside the acknowledgment that autism can have genuinely disabling effects, which are often specific to context. More subtly, this can lead to reflection on the extent to which the "disabling" of autistic persons is a function of the world in which they live, which is constructed around the preferences of the neurotypical. Fourth, one of the dangers with this approach can be that the distinctive abilities of the autistic are celebrated (excellence at certain intellectual tasks, for example) and that this celebration becomes the basis for affirming their value, but in a way that participates in the denigration of those who lack such abilities. Ironically, there can be a kind of "ableism" within the autism community that excludes profoundly autistic persons.

The term "disability," then, may not be as inappropriate as it is sometimes considered to be. If it is embraced, it can itself be addressed in ways that align with disability advocacy: autistic people can speak in quite precise ways about how their condition affects them, and can engage with the conversations around "ableism" in order to challenge discrimination or bias.

Autism and the Church
Identifying Obvious Problems and Opportunities

Before turning to consider the various attempts to define or explain autism, it may be useful to reflect on how the clusters of characteristics above might radically affect the experience of those with autism, and their families, within the environment of the church. This will include the formal services of worship, but also the wider patterns of fellowship. The examples that follow are all real and reflect the testimonies of people with autism or their parents, but they hardly constitute an exhaustive list; plenty of other examples could be mentioned. Mostly they are negative, and it is important to frame them by saying that despite such experiences, autistic people can find churches to be supportive environments where they consider themselves to belong,[22] even while they struggle with certain elements that are personally difficult for them. That said, some have experienced churches as thoroughly hostile places, usually because those in the church do not comprehend the extent to which their environment excludes those with different needs. Readers of this book who are themselves autistic, or who have autistic family members, may well feel that what is described here parallels their experience. They may, with some justification, complain that it actually underplays just how awful their experiences have sometimes been.

There are, of course, lots of different church traditions, with very different practices of worship. Some of the problems are particular to certain traditions, but others straddle the denominational boundaries; readers can, perhaps, map what is described here onto their own church culture and practices. Crucially, in ways that we do not always consider, all churches are sensory and social environments. There will be music (often channeled through a PA system); other people who bring their personal smells and noises into the church; interactions with those people at an informal level of greeting, or perhaps at a formal level within the course of the service; a performance of some kind from the front (sermons and songs, also often channeled through a PA). And there will probably be a social event that follows the service: a busy room with coffee, and people milling about in conversation. Beyond this, the church will probably expect its members to meet at various points during the week, for fellowship events or gatherings, for Bible studies and prayer meetings.

For persons with autism, each of these elements can involve challenges, depending on their particular sensory characteristics. The PA system may not be configured properly, with a whine coming from one of its channels because the wrong cabling has been used or a frequency cutting through because the EQ has not been set properly (note to readers: this will probably be in the 1–2 kHz range, and it really is quite easy to correct), or with that ringing sound that happens when the gain is set too high while the volume faders are sitting too low, or just with the overall volume being too loud. Other people might notice these things, too, but their senses quickly adapt to filter them out. But the person with autism who is sensitive to these noises may not be able to adjust them down or screen them out—they will continue to penetrate for the duration of the service. The effects are exacerbated by the music, as one instrument or voice cuts through, or by the sermon, as the preacher decides that some shouting is required to ram home a point. After the service has finished, someone may start whistling the tune of the closing hymn, or at least attempt to do so; for the person with autism, what comes out of their lips is just a series of high-pitched noises that roughly follows the rhythm of the song. For the person who finds smells difficult, meanwhile, the sanctuary becomes a torture chamber: perfume, cologne, deodorant, hand soap, hair product. It is not simply that these things smell strongly: they smell *painfully*. They smell like a screwdriver being stabbed into the eyes, or the brain being pulled apart.

And, of course, the whole experience is framed by social interactions that are difficult. People greet with handshakes or hugs, with a light touch on the arm that is meant to communicate warmth, but is deeply distressing. People insist on making eye contact, and there are people *everywhere*. During the coffee time afterwards, this is multiplied and intensified. The room is full of threat, because it is filled with people who are communicating in ways that are not easy to understand, coming at the person with autism from all sides. The room is full of subtexts, communicative acts that are spoken in gestures or expressions, or in uses of language that break the rules of the linguistic system. The person with autism is unsure whether they have understood these, and afterwards wonders whether their own contributions were understood properly, or whether they were offensive. They wonder whether they bored that one person to whom they spoke at length about their interests, in the corner away from the crowd. They know that sometimes they can do that, because they don't notice the signs that the person really wants to move on to talk to someone else. They go home exhausted, and perhaps anxious about all of these elements. They cannot face attending a second service that day, or the midweek fellowship group, because they are just too tired. Their senses are raw with exposure, and they are wrecked by the efforts of socializing.

These are the kinds of experiences that adults with autism—whether diagnosed or not—describe. The problems are often even more severe for parents or caregivers of children with autism, or of adults who require ongoing care. The same experiences described above will often translate into behaviors by the child that are difficult for the church community to deal with. In some cases, the child may behave in ways that are so disruptive and difficult that the parent is asked to leave the church.[23] In other cases, particularly when the child is less profoundly affected by autism, they may simply be regarded as strange or unlikable. The child may not socialize with other children the way that one might expect, or may behave in ways that other children and their parents find disconcerting. They may refuse to make eye contact, or may stare. They may openly be described by other parents as unpleasant or even creepy. Where the characteristics of autism are less profound, other parents or members of the church may make it a personal mission to try to "help" the children to fit in and to do what everyone else does.

Often, whether for adults, children, or parents, there is a good deal of judging experienced. Because the perception of boundaries is different, autistic people will be honest in ways that others find unsettling. They will not go along with something simply because it is a convention. They may articulate a view that is considered unthinkable by the community, because they have thought about issues in a very different way, one that is not constrained by the normal instinct to belong. They may be vocal about their distress, or silent in their agreements, feeling no need to join in the cheering. Importantly, in ways that we will explore in the following chapters, they may not be easy people to "like," because so much of what we perceive to be likable in people is linked to their social skills and nonverbal communication. They may be tolerated, but not valued. As we will see, this raises profound questions about our instinct to like certain people: if, as Paul insists, we are constitutionally sinful, with sinful instincts that are woven into our "flesh," then perhaps we need to learn to distrust our intuition to like some people and not others. This will be a significant theme in the chapters that follow: we have to ask whether much of the social dynamic that underpins the unity and community of our churches actually reflects the sinfulness of the people involved. Autism, as we will see, demands that we reconsider this.

In addition, autism can generate a further set of distinctive pastoral needs associated with the wider family. Parents of children with autism need a particular kind of care and support, and may find that their faith assumptions have been challenged in ways that need to be worked through carefully. Spouses of persons with autism, particularly those diagnosed in later life, may have complex emotional needs, wrapped up in the ways that their wife or husband interacts with them. The love of someone with autism for their partner may not manifest itself in ways that are conventional; they may not want to hug or cuddle the partner and may want to spend lengthy times alone. For a spouse who lacks a robust sense of self-confidence, this can be difficult to deal with.

Furthermore, as discussed in chapter 5, autism can often be accompanied by destructive behaviors. Autistic persons can be obsessive about certain things in ways that are difficult for partners or parents; they can also turn to substances for relief from the symptoms of anxiety brought on by sensory difference. Some evidence suggests that those with autism are more vulnerable to addictions than others in the wider population.[24] For pastors, Christian churches, and Christian friends, the pastoral needs around autism can be far-reaching.

Theories and Explanations for the Autism Spectrum

The digression from reviewing research concerning autism into considering its pastoral significance for the church should remind readers that we are not dealing here in abstract theory for its own sake. These issues are very real and very raw for many people, and they are compounded by popular misconceptions about autism, some of which can be traced back to older ways of thinking about the condition that are now obsolete, or at least heavily modified. It is important, then, to provide some kind of review of the accounts and explanations that have been developed for the autism spectrum.

No serious researcher today would advocate a "psychogenic" explanation for autism, where it is understood to be a psychological state generated by poor infant relationships, particularly with the mother. That, however, was how some of the pioneering research into autism framed the condition, and much of the early literature published by Kanner reflected it.[25] Thankfully, better explanations have appeared as research has developed, but there remain popular movements outside of the research community that see autism as something that can be cured by the right kind of interventions or therapies.[26] As we will see in chapter 5, autistic people often learn to adapt their behaviors up to a point, which can be transformational for their lives, but the neurological differences between them and the wider population are not something that can simply be treated with therapy and cured. We are increasingly aware of the plasticity of the human brain and its capacity to be trained and rewired through our practices, but the parameters and limits of this plasticity are determined by the actual structures that are present and their basic configuration. If you are autistic, you are autistic: you may adapt significantly, but you will not stop being autistic.

As research into autism began to develop significantly in the 1980s, when the shift toward understanding it in terms of a spectrum started to take hold, the social and communicative dimension of the condition became the central focus of attention. Researchers drew upon a concept used in psychology called "theory of mind." This is not the same as "philosophy of mind," which is a broad area of philosophical research that seeks to understand what the mind is and how it relates to the world around it. "Theory of mind" (or TOM) is a label that designates the ability of a person or creature to perceive the different cognitive and emotional state of another person or creature. If one "has" a TOM, they can recognize that the other person with whom they interact is in a particular emotional or cognitive state (happy, sad, confused, etc.) and can distinguish that person's state from their own. They are able to ascribe difference to that person's state and to see it as distinct from their own. Some of the psychological research into TOM was concerned to establish whether this ability could be observed in other species than humans, and how it might be related to a concept like personhood.[27] Researchers into autism drew upon this concept, suggesting that persons with autism had a deficient theory of mind, or even lacked a theory of mind entirely. The mechanisms that could explain this deficiency were still unknown, but the core problem was identified as "mind-blindness," a reduced or nonexistent capacity to detect the mental state of another person.[28] In turn, this came to be identified as a deficiency in empathy: since the person with autism could not perceive the state of mind or emotion of the other person, they could not intuitively empathize with them. Autism became seen as a condition of low empathy, a trait that it happened to share with psychopathy.[29]

This basic understanding of autism has underpinned much of the research into the condition and has been explored in relation to what is now often referred to as "the mirror system." This is a component of human neurology that triggers corresponding reactions in a person who sees another person's mental state revealed in the fine grain of their expression and body language. Sometimes people refer to "mirror neurons," but we are really speaking of a whole subsystem within our bodies and brains that fires in sympathy with the firing of neurons in the other person. When a neurotypical person sees a frown, they frown in response, and their psychological state attunes itself to what that frown might betray; when they see a smile, they smile back, and their psychology and emotion shift to a condition of happiness. This mirroring happens all the time and is a key part of the ability to intuitively perceive the emotional state of another person, or to read their nonverbal cues. They may not have spoken any words, but their microgestures, the movements of muscles that have shifted by no more than millimeters, have revealed much about their psychological or emotional state. They have pleaded with their eyes, or shared joy with a crease in their cheek. And the other person has perceived this, without even being consciously aware of it, because their own neurons have fired in sympathy, just as a guitar string will start to buzz when its note is played on another instrument. At least, this is the case if one's mirror system is functioning the way it does in most people. If its function is compromised, then such events of communication will simply not register. This is what is claimed to be the case with autism.

The mirror system is less well understood than is sometimes suggested by the literature.[30] To some extent, discussion of the system involves conjecture based on the study of social and psychological phenomena, rather than neural anatomy. But there is now some evidence that the gross (i.e., nonmicroscopic) neural anatomy of people with autism is different than that of the rest of the population. Their brains, at least in some cases, appear to have different proportions than those considered statistically normal.[31] Various explanations for the differences in development have been considered, one of which we will discuss further below, but genetic factors are clearly high on the list of influences. Autism often crosses generations, even if its manifestation is different in each. Certain genes have already been identified as genomic locations where transcription issues are linked to autism, although autism is probably not associated with a single genetic cause but with a number of genetic factors.

I will say more about the "theory of mind / empathy" explanation below, but I feel that I should offer an observation here about the use of language. Without calling into question the validity of the research itself, or the significance of the mirror system to explanations of autistic behavior, I share the widespread concern within the autism community about the terminological decisions made by researchers. I do not think it is appropriate to label autism as a condition of "low empathy."

For my part, this is because I work all the time with language (actually with multiple languages) and have been sensitized by this to the question of whether words are being used at the right level and with the right significance. To identify a differently developed mirror system with a "lack of empathy" is problematic because the word "empathy" does not designate something that is reducible to the firing of the mirror system. It designates a capacity to perceive the emotional or psychological state of another person and respond appropriately; hence, "empathy" labels something at a higher order than physiology. The autistic person whose mirror system is not triggered by the manifest suffering of another person may still arrive at a perception of that person's pain by a different pathway; they may have acquired experience that allows them to know that the person is, for example, grieving, and they may reach to offer the kind of comfort that they have learned is expected. To describe them as "lacking empathy" is simply to confuse an interpretive phenomenon of perception with *one* of the mechanisms by which it can be attained.[32]

Similarly, to say that a person with autism has no theory of mind is potentially offensive and misleading: it implies that they do not recognize the presence of a neurological state in another person that is different than that in themselves. In truth, however, autistic people do recognize this. They simply need different means to actually understand that state than the intuitive ones that others enjoy. Many within the autism community are understandably hostile to being labeled as having low empathy or deficient theory of mind, since the natural implication of such labeling is that they do not care about others and are incapable of showing love and compassion. Researchers may protest that their use of the language has been taken out of context and not understood as they intended, but they should be open to recognizing that their choice of terminology may be intrinsically problematic within the system of language itself. Put bluntly, when autism researchers use the word "empathy," they do not mean what the word itself means. That suggests to me that a different word should be used.

I need to stress, however, that this is a comment on terminology, rather than on the underlying research. That research has also suggested that persons with autism have a high systematizing tendency: they are drawn to systems, perceive systems, and often impose systems. The Autism Research Centre at the University of Cambridge has mapped the systematizing tendency of persons with autism and correlated it with what tend to be labeled "low empathy scores": they consider these measurable and have devised tests to measure the systematizing and empathizing "quotients" of the individual, which can be factored into an "autism quotient." This was the basis for a massive online study that used the autism quotient questionnaire, which resulted in some of the assumptions of autism research (particularly concerning gender spread) being challenged.[33]

Those associated with this approach have compared the "high systematizing, low empathizing" quotients of persons with the general population, differentiating male and female scores. They have argued that the scores seen in persons with autism look like a more extreme version of the general differences between males and females, even labeling autism as a kind of extreme male brain. This has not gone without challenge, and it is important to note that the theory was developed at a time when autism was believed to be present principally among males, with only a small number of females affected. That is no longer believed to be the case. Autism is now believed to affect both equally, but simply to be underreported or better camouflaged among females.[34]

Some more recent studies have focused on the sensory features of autism. While it is unlikely that the sensory dimension stands as a sole cause of all of the presenting features of autism, several scholars have moved it from the periphery of the discussion—as if it were merely a quirky side-effect of the condition—to the center.[35] This is reflected in diagnostic approaches to autism, which increasingly focus on the distinctive sensory issues as indicative that the person is indeed autistic. It is likely that the sensory issues are a function of the differences in neural proportion and connectivity that lead to the other symptoms of autism. As mentioned already, it is not that the sensory receptors themselves are any more sensitive than they are in members of the wider population, but rather that the brain's filtering and interpretive mechanisms do not work in the same way. We tend to assume that that the information that passes through our senses into our brains creates a sensory picture of the world as it actually is, so that what we see, hear, smell, taste, and feel corresponds exactly to what is around us. Actually, our brains are constantly filtering the flow of sensory information, dropping unimportant data from the picture we form and interpreting the data that come in. Recently, various online "memes" have highlighted the extent to which we do this, such as pictures of strawberries that are rendered in grayscale but are "seen" in color. For autistic people, the filters appear to work differently, and the interpretation can be quite different. Where a "normal" person will quickly stop perceiving a fragrance (which they might find quite pleasant), a person with autism may be unable to screen it out. Colors can be more densely saturated for someone with autism, to the extent that their brain can be overwhelmed by the intensity of the colorscape through which they are moving. Again, where the typical person will only notice sounds that their brain considers important, the person with autism might be flooded with the information about every sound detectable in their space, whether loud or quiet. While trying to converse with someone, they may also hear the whine of electrical items, the sound of someone munching potato chips nearby, someone whistling in the street, a mouse scratching in the walls, or something else that is quiet but insistent and that they desperately need to identify. Their perceptions of the world may, in fact, be much more authentic as sensory pictures of the world than those of the typical person, since they may be less filtered or less heavily interpreted (although it should be stressed that the filtering process may also be different, rather than diminished). Authentic is not the same as useful, though. Sometimes the volume of detail that is vivid in the brain of the person with autism leads to sensory overload: there are too many things for the person to deal with or to screen out, and their brain can no longer process it. They may resort to stimming behavior at this point, as a reflexive way of creating security in the midst of the sensory torment, or they may have a "meltdown." Some of the destructive behavior seen in profoundly autistic persons may be a result of such sensory overload, which they cannot verbalize.

Vaccines and Autism

A Dangerous Fraud

One last explanation for autism needs to be mentioned here because it continues to be held in some popular circles and is supported by a particular subculture. This explanation has linked autism to vaccine programs, particularly those involving complex vaccines such as MMR. The claim, at its heart, is that the vaccines compromise the lining of the gut, leading to inflammation and malabsorption, which in turn leads to the neurological problems that present as autism. The "research" that underpins this claim was published in an eminent medical journal, *The Lancet*, but was subsequently withdrawn from the journal—its publication status revoked—as its methodology was demonstrated to be problematic and as multiple conflicts of interest came to light in relation to its principal author, Andrew Wakefield.[36] What had initially appeared to be a credible research article was subsequently demonstrated to have manipulated and misrepresented data in ways that were considered unethical given the (undisclosed) funding that had paid for the study, which represented vested interests.[37] This point needs to be stated with as much force as possible: the scientific merit of the study has been conclusively falsified.

The media publicity that the study was given, however, caused it to be widely influential, and after Wakefield was struck off the medical register in the UK for professional misconduct, he began to publish his claims in more popular, and less rigorously evaluated, contexts.[38] There continues to be a movement that seeks to link the surge in numbers of children presenting with autism symptoms to vaccination programs, particularly those involving complex vaccines. As is typically the case with such movements, they are fed by valid observations (e.g., there is some evidence that persons with autism are more commonly affected by gut disorders) that become the basis for nonvalid conclusions (that those gut disorders caused the autism in the first place, and were themselves caused by vaccines). We might hope that they will eventually give way to the growing body of evidence for genetic causes, which can be traced back far beyond the point when a vaccine is administered, but the present time is famously one in which the scientific community is treated with mistrust and conspiracy theories run amok, empowered by social media, in which prominent individuals have a strong presence. Christian communities are often particularly influenced by those theories, which means that there is a high likelihood that Christians will be forced to engage with them and may have been unhelpfully directed by them.

Conclusion

In this chapter, I have sought to provide as up-to-date an overview of autism and its symptoms as possible. The research into autism develops apace, and the theories and explanatory accounts are constantly being modified. Those who want to remain abreast of such developments should make use of the websites associated with the various autistic societies and may want to establish connections with local branches.

The most important point to be stressed in the discussion above is that autism does not "go away," any more than Down syndrome goes away. It is a lifelong condition that means the persons in question will perceive and experience the world in ways that are nontypical. This creates a distinctive set of needs, for the individual person with autism and for those around them. These may change through the life experience of the person, but they will never vanish. The experiences and associated needs may range from subtle to severe: autism may be a "hidden disability" that leads to the person being misunderstood in specific ways by those around them, or it may be visibly profound in its effects, leaving the person in need of lifelong care.

This diversity—the complexity that is labeled by the term "autism spectrum"—needs to be kept in view throughout what follows. Some parts of the discussion will bear particularly on those who are profoundly affected by autism, to the extent of needing lifelong care, while other parts will bear on those who would never have been diagnosed as autistic in previous generations. With autism, it is difficult (and often impossible) to generalize, and readers will need to be prepared to apply the discussion that follows in later chapters in variegated and differentiated ways. This demands, too, that our evaluation of autism be appropriately nuanced and variegated. Much of the theological engagement with autism rightly seeks to give a positive account of the condition and its place within the church, but we cannot allow this to blind us to the real difficulties and suffering that it can often bring. We have to develop ways of speaking about autism that allow us to identify certain of its elements or aspects as *bad*,[39] without thereby labeling the condition in wholly negative terms.

Reflecting on the different experiences of those with autism requires us to think about what is taken for granted within our own experience, or what is assumed to be "normal." One of the key themes in disability studies, particularly those interested in operating theologically, is the extent to which "normality" (or "normalcy") can reflect social constructs, values, or assumptions that need to be challenged. The relevance of this to the lived experience of autism within the church is obvious. At the same time, some theological study makes use of autism precisely as it exemplifies "abnormality" or deficiency and uses it as a contrast to what normal life within God's world *should* look like.[40]

Personally, I find this *essentially negative* approach to autism troubling, and the next two chapters will involve some reflection on whether it is a biblically defensible treatment of autism.

As we turn to consider the biblical material that might inform our Christian thinking on autism, one of the key themes that will emerge is precisely that our sinfulness and constitutional idolatry often manifest themselves in a set of presumed values that are held to account by God. Such values often center on what (or whom) we perceive to be strong or weak, valuable or worthless. They also center on how our categories of difference tacitly shape the way we think about inclusion and exclusion, or about belonging, or about status within the community. Importantly, those values are necessarily subject to reevaluation once we identify our object of worship with a Galilean peasant who dies a violent death as a convicted criminal, incapacitated and then terminated by wounds that continue to be visible in his risen flesh. Once this man is worshiped as the Creator and Sustainer of all things, our ethical world is entirely redrawn.

2

AUTISM AND THE BIBLE
The Challenge of Reading Responsibly

Your word is a lamp to my feet and a light to my path.
—Psalm 119:105

This chapter is intended as a programmatic summary of the approach to reading the Bible that will be taken in this book. We are, of course, concerned with an issue that was not known or named as such in the ancient world and is nowhere explicitly described in Scripture. We cannot, then, simply find several relevant passages and engage in exegesis, after which we pronounce, "This is what the Bible says about autism." We need to think more carefully about how the Bible, considered as the normative and sacred Scripture of the Christian tradition, should function to shape our thinking about autism. This, in fact, is a principle of understanding how biblical authority operates that extends beyond the particulars of autism to a massive range of uniquely modern issues. The world is full of things that were unknown to our parents, far less to the biblical authors, and one of the constant dangers that besets Christians who rightly consider the Bible to regulate their thought and life is of moving to facile assumptions about how these ancient texts might speak to contemporary realities. This speaks, in turn, to the simplistic ways in which we often apply texts that do refer clearly to a particular issue to contemporary ethics: we often move immediately from the exegesis of this or that text to a pronouncement on the rights or wrongs of a particular practice. The problem with this is that it often neglects something that was a vital interpretive principle for the early church, the question of how any given text is to be read within the context of the Bible as a whole, and in relation to the gospel of Jesus Christ. While this principle, known as "the rule of faith" (*regula fidei*), developed fluidly and without much explicit articulation, it was widely sustained.[1] The commitment to relating the exegesis of any given passage to the canon as a whole and to the person of Jesus Christ reflected an important recognition: the Bible can be *misused* in the service of ideology, and our interpretations of it must be undertaken carefully and prayerfully. Most of the views that the church has come to label as heresy have been based upon "proof texts," from which the proponents of those views have claimed biblical warrant. As we seek to think Christianly about autism, we may find ourselves reconsidering what it means think Christianly at all, and how the Bible operates within this.

The principles that I lay out here are drawn from some of my own recent work on Christian moral identity and on Christian intellectual humility,[2] both of which have been particularly attentive to how the Bible functions to shape the way that we think. They are also influenced by my involvement with discussions about the theology of disability. I currently teach at the University of Aberdeen, in my home country of Scotland; one of the distinctive features of our department is a particular interest in theology and disability, represented in the work of my wonderful colleagues John Swinton and Brian Brock, who have thought much longer and much harder than I have about disability (a word that we use out of necessity, rather than preference), and whose thinking has been shaped at the most basic levels by personal experience. To work within an academic community where disability is of central concern is a privilege, and it forces one to consider many of the interpretive values that we take for granted and ask whether they are problematic at a deep level. The principles I outline here have been shaped by this context; they are not uniquely about autism, or even disability more broadly, but about the ways that we basically conceive the task of reading Scripture. They bear on every issue that we might consider, not just the one that is our principal burden in this book. Consequently, they may invite readers to reconsider their views on a whole range of issues beyond the current one. But I offer them here because they are absolutely vital to a proper use of the Bible in relation to the needs of those with autism. As I indicated in the previous chapter, reflecting Christianly on autism may press us to reevaluate the basic assumptions that govern our practices, even those of exegesis. It may cause us to see that our cherished readings of Scripture are actually idolatrous or vicious. This is something that each reader can consider for him- or herself. Here, I simply offer a set of programmatic statements that take their own authority from the character of Scripture itself and from the interpretive principles that can be traced back to the earliest Christians, the church fathers who left us a legacy of christological and Trinitarian doctrine.

Before I do this, though, I will consider three examples of trying to think biblically about autism that I consider to be fundamentally flawed. Identifying the flaws in each will allow us to think a little more maturely about how the Bible should function properly in our theology.

Misreading the Bible in Relation to Autism

The first example is, on one level, fairly innocuous, but it still opens up some important issues for us to reflect upon. In a 2010 article, S. K. Mathew and J. D. Pandian "diagnosed" a number of biblical characters as having what are known today to be neurological or psychiatric conditions.[3] Among the characters they diagnosed was Samson, whom they considered to be autistic; this "would precede the first known case of autism by centuries."[4] Without needing to rehearse any of the detail behind this proposed diagnosis, we can compare Mathew and Pandian's approach with the process of clinical diagnosis that would be experienced by a person with autism today. This involves lengthy interviews, both with the person (if they are able to communicate) and with family members. A detailed picture of their background and development is constructed, shaped (as far as possible) by the person's own testimony concerning their sensory and social experiences. The process may take more than one day of interviews, and is regulated by very detailed, carefully developed questions of agreed diagnostic value. It is simply impossible to replicate this by relying on the limited third-person narrative detail of a biblical story contained in four short chapters of the Bible. (As an aside, I might note the parallels with the kind of "diagnosis" often passed by church members or pastors on other members of the congregation whom they consider to be "on the spectrum." This is usually a dismissive diagnosis, based, again, on an inadequate body of specific evidence.)

The approach also engages with the biblical story as a means to access a historical reality that lies behind the text and is obtainable through it; that is, the principal thing that the authors are seeking to obtain through their reading of the text is access to the historical reality of Samson's neurotype. Doing so neglects the real character, function, and purpose of the narrative and the discourse, which is to *communicate* to its readers something that will shape their own lives in relation to God. This is not to question the historical veracity of the text—that is a debate for elsewhere—but to emphasize that the text is not principally intended as a vehicle for historical documentation, but rather for edification. As such, whatever historical details the text contains are rendered to us in a theological and edificational narrative that is much more concerned with the demands of Yahwism and the dangers of idolatry than with the neurological health of its characters.[5] Put bluntly, Mathew and Pandian's approach to the text of the book of Judges is not appropriate to the character of the text.

The second example is dramatically more disturbing, to the extent that I feel the need to issue a trigger warning to any parents of profoundly autistic children that what follows may be upsetting. I am also sufficiently disturbed by it that I do not want to publish a link to the relevant websites, since I do not want to promote them in any sense. In the course of my research, I came across a website that compared the symptoms of autism (actually profound autism, although no such differentiation was made in the discussion itself) to the biblical accounts of demon possession. Mutism, fits, spasms, destructive behavior, and so on: these were represented as significant parallels between the descriptions in the Gospels of people who had demons driven from them and the behaviors seen in autistic children. The conclusion reached was that what is seen as an epidemic of autism today is actually evidence of demon possession. The correct way to treat this, therefore, is with prayers for deliverance or exorcism. As disturbing as this claim was in itself, it was overshadowed by the comments that readers had posted to the website about their own experience as parents. They affirmed the identification of autism with demon possession and, in many cases, spoke about their own experience of praying (unsuccessfully) for their own children to be delivered from the demons that possessed them.

Multiple responses could be made to this; these will be reprised in the positive proposals outlined below. For one thing, stories of demonic possession within the Bible are actually relatively uncommon and are particularly clustered within the Synoptic Gospels and Acts. There are only a few stories outside these. That fact has some bearing on the proportional significance of the demonic within the Bible and relates to one of the proposals below, namely that we need to allow biblical proportions to play some role in our biblical interpretation, to respect the shape of the Bible as a whole. Second, the association of a demonic presence with a nonverbal (mute) person is really confined to two stories (Matt 9:32-33 / Luke 11:14; Matt 12:22); only by conflating these stories with others involving demons and violence (Matt 8:28-33) can one construct something that shares superficial characteristics with autism. Third, "mutism" or "nonverbalism" is more commonly represented in the Bible simply as a physical disability, listed alongside lameness and blindness as people come to Jesus for healing (about which we will say more below), as in Matthew 15:30-31. The final point is perhaps the most important: the problem with this approach is that it does not take seriously the need to understand what we are bringing *back* to the Bible to be understood in its light. It ignores the evidence that autism is associated with genetic factors and with demonstrably different neurological features; it does not take seriously enough that these are necessarily part of what the condition is and involves. Those who contributed to the website mentioned above might accuse me here of putting modern science "before" the Bible, but it is actually a basic principle of biblical truthfulness that we expect to see a coherence between the physical world that science investigates and the world as it is rendered to us in Scripture. The two involve different identifications and therefore different principles of investigation,[6] and they cannot be collapsed into each other, but we expect to see some kind of coherence, of a kind that means we cannot ignore the physical dimension of autism (genetics, neurology, etc.) by labeling it as demon possession. I will say more below on how we negotiate the technological present in relation to the pretechnological past, but at this point the main problem with this approach can be expressed in these terms: its advocates do not take seriously the evidence for the physical causal factors known to be associated with autism.[7]

The third problematic use of the Bible is more subtly wrong, although it may be nearly as disturbing as the one just considered. For some, autism is a problem to be "healed." This view takes its warrant from the various stories of healing that we find in the Bible, particularly in the New Testament, and most extensively within the context of the Gospels and Acts. In some cases, it can be married to what is sometimes referred to as a "health and prosperity" understanding of the gospel, where those who have true faith in God enjoy a flood of blessings that ought typically to include the healing of illnesses and the provision of material prosperity. Sometimes this is traced to a view of sickness and suffering that links them very closely to the problem of sin: where sin is properly dealt with, healing and prosperity should follow. For reasons that I will outline below, this approach should be seen as highly problematic. In other cases, though, the view of where healing and blessing fit into Christian experience may be less sweeping and less thoroughly problematic: they may be affirmed as things that often, but not always, accompany God's life-giving presence, to be prayed for and hoped for, but not considered to be routine.

Any reflection on this must affirm that the Bible includes stories of healing, sometimes involving people who are disabled in some sense. It must also recognize that some of those healings appear to have a programmatic significance, representing the decisive change that has taken place with the coming of Jesus and closely linked to the realization of his work of deliverance from sin. In Matthew 11, for example, Jesus responds to John's question about whether he is indeed the Messiah in part by referring to his work of healing:

> ² When John heard in prison what the Messiah was doing, he sent word by his disciples ³ and said to him, "Are you the one who is to come, or are we to wait for another?" ⁴ Jesus answered them, "Go and tell John what you hear and see: ⁵ the blind receive their sight, the lame walk, the lepers are cleansed, the deaf hear, the dead are raised, and the poor have good news brought to them. ⁶ And blessed is anyone who takes no offense at me." (Matt 11:2-6)

The references to those who are healed are generally understood to evoke the expectations of the prophet Isaiah about the figure of the Servant, so that their function is not to indicate that healing will now be the new normal, but rather to demonstrate that Jesus is, indeed, the messianic Servant. This is in line with other parts of Matthew that similarly link the revelation of the Davidic king with particular acts of healing.[8] Nevertheless, the healings are described as real events, and we should take this seriously. We must also acknowledge that there are points in the Bible, notably in the Psalms,[9] where the language of sickness and affliction is used by people who are burdened by a sense of their own sin, and who identify their suffering as some kind of divine chastening.

These observations mean that we cannot ignore the *apparent* biblical warrant for the view that autism, like any other disabling condition, might be (or even "should be") healed. But the same can be said of every view that, through the centuries, the church has come to consider wrong or even heretical: all can point to particular scriptural texts for warrant. The proper response to these must always be to highlight that other parts of the canon of Scripture contain important corrective or balancing truths that

must be brought to bear on such assertions. In relation to healing in general, it needs to be noted that the stories of healing,
as with those concerning exorcism, are particularly clustered
within the Gospels and Acts, where they continue to have an
exceptional significance. The miracles of Jesus continued to be
"miraculous" and not commonplace; they are exceptional interventions, rather than the norm. The same is true of the miracles
in Acts: only a small number of healings stories are recounted,
which must be considered *exceptionally significant*. James, certainly, speaks of the prayer offered in faith that will make the
sick person well (5:15), and does so in a way that suggests he is
speaking about regular practices of prayer, but his words need
to be read alongside the passages in Paul's writings that speak
of suffering and sickness as things that continue to be present in
the life of the believer and that are vital to our manifestation of
divine grace:

> [7] But we have this treasure in clay jars, so that it may be made
> clear that this extraordinary power belongs to God and does
> not come from us. [8] We are afflicted in every way, but not
> crushed; perplexed, but not driven to despair; [9] persecuted,
> but not forsaken; struck down, but not destroyed; [10] always
> carrying in the body the death of Jesus, so that the life of
> Jesus may also be made visible in our bodies. (2 Cor 4:7-10)

This leads toward one of the core principles that must inform
the use of Scripture, which simply recognizes that any given
text or passage needs to be considered within the wider context of the Bible as a whole. One of the most basic problems
in contemporary Christian uses of Scripture is a tendency to
move immediately from the exegesis of an isolated text (or even
a small set of texts) to making a moral or theological claim that
is asserted as "biblical." This problem becomes visible quickly
when we seek to deal with an issue like autism, but it affects
our moral and theological reasoning much more broadly. As we

will see below, such an approach fails to show proper respect or reverence to the character of Scripture as a complex work of divine communication.

One further point can be made on the topic of healing and on the use of Scripture in relation to it. As readers, we need to be sensitive to the ways in which our basic assumptions are colored by the social and intellectual context of late modernity, and we need to allow Scripture to challenge those assumptions. One of the subtle issues that we face concerns our perception of what it means to be healthy and whole. Within the modern context—in which we have come to cherish the idea of the self-contained, self-reliant, autonomous individual[10]—we tend to think of health and well-being in individualist terms, assuming that the healthy individual is one who needs no care and who can live a productive and constructive life. We may even map the need for care and support onto a theology in which the image of God has been compromised and damaged by sin.[11]

Without necessarily dismissing this view, we need to be open to the possibility that we are refracting the biblical material through a distinctively modern account of human being, which neglects the possibility that one can live a joyful life of flourishing while being entirely dependent on the caregiving of others.[12] Often this accompanies a particular conception of the image of God (*imago Dei*), one that links it to the possession and manifestation of certain properties or capacities by the individual. Such an understanding can be traced back into premodern theology, but it becomes radically more dominant in the modern era, in the wake of the Enlightenment and the influence of humanism. At this stage, I am not seeking to offer an alternative way of thinking about the *imago Dei*, but simply to alert the reader to the possibility that they may be working with a set of very modern assumptions about what it means to be a flourishing human being, and may think of healing (and, for that matter, our ultimately destined condition) in ways that are shaped by this.

The problems with both of these approaches—the identification of autism as demonic and the expectation that it should be healed—are complex, but generally emerge from a tendency to read certain biblical passages without due consideration for the teaching of the wider Bible, rather than from misreading the passages in themselves. The principles offered in what follows will, I hope, provide helpful correctives to this.

Principle 1: We Read the Bible in a Way That Is Governed by the Person and Story of Jesus Christ

To read the Bible "Christianly" means to read all of the Bible in a way that is informed and governed by the identity of Jesus Christ, "the mystery that has been hidden throughout the ages and generations but has now been revealed to his saints" (Col 1:26). He is the Word that became flesh (John 1:14), and John's identification of him in such terms is suggestive of the fact that the meaning of Scripture must always be approached through his particular embodiment of it; for, as John continues, "no one has ever seen God; it is God the Only Begotten, who is in the Father's heart, who has made him known" (John 1:18, my translation).

To say this should be fairly uncontroversial to any Christian reader, but its importance can be attenuated by ways of conceiving "Christ-centeredness" that fall short of the way it is rendered in the New Testament. It is not simply that Jesus is the great exemplar of Christian morality, whose behavior is to be emulated and whose lead is to be followed; neither is it simply the case that Jesus is now identified as the God to whom obedience is rendered. In the first, Christ-centeredness is a matter of imitation (exemplified in the "What would Jesus do?" slogan), while in the second it is a matter of worshipful obedience to the king. Both of these are good and important elements of Christ-centeredness, but taken by themselves they fall short of the way that the New Testament writers speak of Christ, not just as one by whom obedience is modeled, or to whom it is rendered, but as the one *in* whom salvation and goodness are constituted, and apart from whom they do not exist. This language is ubiquitous in Paul's writing, but it is found widely through the New Testament. The words of Jesus that are reported in John's Gospel communicate the significance of the incorporative grammar most effectively: "Those who abide in me and I in them bear much fruit, because apart from me you can do nothing" (John 15:5).

Importantly, at several points in the New Testament, this kind of language is used both of salvation and of creation, or even of God's providential care for the cosmos. In Colossians 1:15-20, for example, Paul writes:[13]

> [15] He is the image of the invisible God, the firstborn of all creation; [16] for in him all things in heaven and on earth were created, things visible and invisible, whether thrones or dominions or rulers or powers—all things have been created through him and for him. [17] He himself is before all things, and in him all things hold together. [18] He is the head of the body, the church; he is the beginning, the firstborn from the dead, so that he might come to have first place in everything. [19] For in him all the fullness of God was pleased to dwell, [20] and through him God was pleased to reconcile to himself all things, whether on earth or in heaven, by making peace through the blood of his cross. (Col 1:15-20)

Here it is not only salvation that is "in Christ," as it is often represented in Paul's writings, but everything in creation, from before time and into eternity. They are not, of course, all "in" him in the same way,[14] but the text is particularly concerned to highlight the corresponding senses in which creation, providence, and redemption are constituted in and through the person of Jesus Christ. When the text goes on to speak of him as the mystery that had been hidden through the ages but has now been revealed (1:26), this is more than just a reference to the importance of the events narrated in the gospel as part of God's unfolding plan of redemption: it is, instead, an articulation of the new perception that the entirety of God's dealings with the cosmos throughout its existence has been done "in Christ." The reading of any text of the Old Testament, then, must now be conditioned for the Christian by the knowledge of who Jesus Christ is.

This is illustrated by what we see in the opening of John's Gospel, where Jesus (represented as "the Word") is described as the one who made all things and in whom the light that gives life to all things exists:

> ³ All things came into being through him, and without him not one thing came into being. What has come into being ⁴ in him was life, and the life was the light of all people. (John 1:3-4)

This is often read as if John is simply using creation imagery to render the identity of Jesus; he is doing this, but he is also retelling the story of creation in christological terms. The imagery in John 1 draws upon both the account of Genesis 1 and the description of Wisdom in Proverbs 8, but the force of the appropriation is to recast both creation and the enjoyment of God's life-giving presence as inseparable from the person of Jesus Christ. When, later in the Gospel, Jesus tells his disciples that "apart from me you can do nothing" (John 15:5), he is not speaking principally as moral exemplar, but as the source of goodness itself.

Grappling with this involves some reflection on notions of "participation." If these passages are taken seriously, then all goodness involves some kind of participation in the life of God through Jesus Christ, even if we necessarily distinguish the kind of participation that is experienced by the believer from the kind that might be embodied by any person or creature that does or enjoys good. This was one of the key themes in the writings of the early church fathers, who recognized that all goodness is derived from the presence of Jesus Christ, but were also concerned to affirm the special kind of participation that is involved in salvation, and that is enjoyed by those who believe and partake of the sacraments.[15]

This is important because it presses back on a way of reading the Bible that reduces the gospel to a "fix" for the problem of sin, a correction of the damage introduced by the fall. Instead, it demands that we read all of the Bible as "evangelically conditioned" and oriented toward a particular kind of flourishing, when God will be all in all (1 Cor 15:28) and will bring each creature to its telos. The ramifications of this point will be very significant when we move into the substance of the following chapters and will have a particular bearing on how we think about the image of God.

Principle 2: We Read the Bible as a Complex Whole

The Bible, considered as holy Scripture, is normative for the thought and life of the Christian church, but it exercises this normativity as a generically diverse collection or even as a library. This is simply a matter of observing and acknowledging that our sacred Scriptures contain poems, proverbs, stories, songs, sayings, prophecies, letters, and some commandments. Certain parts of the collection may have a particular programmatic significance for other parts (the Gospel narratives, most obviously), but one of the problems that needs to be challenged is the tendency to think of "biblical authority" in a way that is reduced to one or two of the genres. The point has been made by David Kelsey and reiterated by Kevin Vanhoozer, and it is worth pausing to reflect on the observations that they have made.[16]

When we think of "biblical authority," we tend to allow one or two particular concepts to govern our ways of thinking, most commonly that of the commandment that should be obeyed or of the reliable account of salvation history within which we understand ourselves. Importantly, those concepts tend to be accompanied by a particular governing metaphor about God's relationship to us: he is seen as the legislator (or king) who, through the biblical salvation history, creates the world and then brings it back into order when sin makes it go wrong by the breaking of his commandments. This feeds into our understanding of gospel and atonement, which are principally conceived in terms of a kind of debt collection for our failure to keep the commandments.[17] As a result, we often think of the Bible as a "manual for life" and conceive its authority in ways that reflect this, while reducing salvation to the notion that commandment breakers are delivered from the punishment that they deserve.

This concept of authority, however, struggles to accommodate many of the genres of Scripture and the way that they operate. It is not easy to apply it to the mode of normativity exercised by the book of Proverbs, which rattles off saying after saying informed by the kind of wisdom that comes from long observation of the world, from lessons learned by watching ants work and vicious people plot. Neither does it easily accommodate the normativity of a psalm, or even, for that matter, of a short story that does not obviously or significantly take forward the grand scheme of salvation history. It may not deal meaningfully with the storied character of the Gospels and Acts, the way that they shape our thinking *as narratives*,[18] and may squeeze their material into an account of "the gospel" or "salvation history" that is actually abstracted from much of the detail.

We need to recognize that Scripture *norms* and *regulates* our life and thought as a wild and unruly collection of works.[19] This involves a certain humility, an acknowledgment that we will never master or own it, but will instead subject ourselves to its abrasion, by reading it and allowing its wordplay to affect us as readers. Like all literature, it does this by engaging us holistically, by shaping our affections and sympathies as much as our propositional beliefs. It shapes us as a library.[20]

Recognizing this prevents us from approaching scriptural authority as something that can be reduced to proof texts for a particular position. All texts need to be evaluated within the context of the collection as a whole, which involves thinking about how other generic parts of the Bible might inform, correct, or nuance what is suggested by the text in front of us. If this sounds worryingly open and unresolved, it should: we should be unnerved by our reading of Scripture; our assumptions should be challenged by it.[21] There are certainly truths that can be seen as necessary to Christian faith, but even these have generally been distilled into doctrines that take seriously the whole of Scripture; there are no proof texts for the Trinity, but Trinitarianism is the correct doctrinal formulation of what the Bible, *as a whole*, teaches us about God.

In relation to our discussion of autism, the point is vital, and it takes us back to the misuses of Scripture discussed above. These focus on a particular set of texts that speak about demonic realities or healings, but do not frame these in relation to the biblical texts that represent sickness or weakness as conditions in which grace can truly flourish, as necessary elements of our participation in the witness of Jesus Christ. Instead, this approach directs us toward a reflection on broader principles that can be traced across the genres of Scripture and that emerge in the complex moral account reflected in the Old Testament, both in the Law and in the wisdom writings. These have a scope and a level of practical detail that is not seen in the New Testament, but is arguably assumed by the various writers. The Law regulates religious life and the festal calendar, but it also regulates agricultural and architectural principles; it bears on worship, but it also bears on social justice and wealth distribution. It bears on the way that a society values its members, both human and animal, especially those who are vulnerable. This is the kind of detailed picture in which we can begin to think about autism and Christian community.

Principle 3: We Respect the Historical Particularities of the Bible

This third principle is worded with special care. Most biblical scholars recognize the importance of engaging with the biblical texts as historical documents, so that some engagement with their historical context or background is necessary to their interpretation. To a significant extent, however, this part of the biblical scholarly task has come to dominate the conception of the task as a whole, so that the majority of serious biblical scholars now effectively work as historians rather than theologians. This is one of the reasons why so little has been done to address the question of how we should think biblically about disabilities that are not encountered in ancient biblical texts: if biblical scholars cannot find historical data in the text or its background that correspond to a contemporary topic, they will have nothing to say to it. In relation to autism, the only way we can escape this is by recovering a properly theological vision for the task. Reading the Bible properly summons us to speak rightly of God, and speaking rightly of God forces us to speak differently about everything else.

But it remains the case that the biblical texts are historically particular and took their form through the organic agency of historically located persons,[22] even if these persons were inspired by the Spirit to communicative acts that continue to speak throughout the ages. It is necessary to acknowledge this in our attempts to read the Bible, and to remind ourselves constantly that we read the texts as cultural foreigners to the worlds in which they were written.[23] The danger that attends us is always that we see something in the text that is not there (or, conversely, that we fail to see something that *is* there). If we read the Bible carefully, sensitive to this, then the world of the text can reach forward to ours, absorbing and reshaping it, investing it with fresh value. If we read it carelessly, we will absorb the world of the text to ours, smothering its radical qualities with our conventional ones.

An example of this is found in the issue of gender roles. In the modern West, we live in a world that has dramatically reordered the respective status of males and females. Many Christians, of course, consider this to be a rejection of biblical gender roles and rail against it. That very reaction, though, often reflects a lack of recognition of just how radical the cultural shift that has taken place within the New Testament Christian community is, and how far it has already gone toward reordering perceptions of the value and role of women. Many Christians today will understand the Bible to reflect their own ecclesial situation, in which men and women play different roles and functionally have different value; they will point to texts in the New Testament that seem to reflect this complementarian structure.[24] They will generally, though, not recognize the historical sociological significance attached to the fact that a church meets in the home of a woman—which would assign her a position of leadership and oversight—or the fact that Paul, departing spectacularly from the conventions of the day, will direct his commendations and greetings to named women within the church in Rome. Those familiar with the culture of the day and the way it ascribed honor and status according to gender are right to see something quite subversive in Romans 16:

> [1] I commend to you our sister Phoebe, a deacon of the church at Cenchreae, [2] so that you may welcome her in the Lord as is fitting for the saints, and help her in whatever she may

require from you, for she has been a benefactor of many and of myself as well. ³ Greet Prisca and Aquila, who work with me in Christ Jesus, ⁴ and who risked their necks for my life, to whom not only I give thanks, but also all the churches of the Gentiles. ⁵ Greet also the church in their house. Greet my beloved Epaenetus, who was the first convert in Asia for Christ. ⁶ Greet Mary, who has worked very hard among you. ⁷ Greet Andronicus and Junia, my relatives who were in prison with me; they are prominent among the apostles, and they were in Christ before I was. (Rom 16:1-7)

The reason for citing this passage is simply that its shocking power is only appreciated if the reader knows something about the cultural conventions of the day and the sociological force of its departures from these. To describe Phoebe as a benefactor (or "patron") is to label her as a person of power, to ascribe honor and authority to her. To describe the church as meeting in the house of Prisca *and* Aquila is to assign ownership of the house to both of them, a fundamentally antipatriarchal move. When we come to consider how the biblical material might bear on autism, the cultural subversiveness of the text, understood within its historical context, will also be an important element, particularly in our reading of 1 Corinthians (see chapter 3).

That said, an important corollary of respecting the historical particularity of the text is that we recognize the extent to which the authors might have thought about disability or impairments in ways that we find difficult or even unacceptable. We need to accept that the Bible is full of stories that reflect the social stigmatizing of persons with disabilities of various kinds and that the authors may have regarded these in ways that were woven into their culture.²⁵ We should not try to minimize or downplay the significance of such elements, but we should also recognize that they reflect the organic inspiration of Scripture and the involvement of human writers whose own contributions are transformed by the canonical context into which they are assembled. Again, the recognition that we read the whole canon in the light of what has been disclosed in the person of Jesus Christ is absolutely pivotal to the right handling of such observations: now that we know this truth, we cannot consider any of the parts of the Bible apart from it. It is a transformational context.

Principle 4: We Read the Bible within the Communion of the Church

There is an irreducibly social dimension to the life governed by scriptural authority. Scripture is directed toward reading communities who engage with the material in the context of communal practice and life. In fact, for most believers until relatively recently (and still for many outside of the developed world), the only way that Scripture could be encountered was socially, because most Christians were illiterate and were therefore reliant on others to read it to (or with) them. Some may have been fortunate to have had literate parents, but most would encounter Scripture primarily in the context of worship, where it was read within the performance of praise and sacrament.

In the context of the developed West and global North, where literacy rates are high and where (as we have already noted) a certain individualism is basically assumed, this social dimension can be undervalued or neglected. Reading and listening to the Bible can be "privatized" into something that the individual does within their personal walk of faith, even if they associate themselves with a church community. *I* ask what moral burden the text lays on *me*, rather than on *us*, and the social or corporate dimension of the church follows this, as an obligation that devolves first upon me. *I* align myself with a particular church community because it holds views to which *I* subscribe. Even the notion of church unity becomes a function of the collective agreement of a group of individuals to a set of beliefs or practices; it is defined in voluntarist terms.

Ironically, our personal reading can actually be very heavily conditioned by the way the Bible is understood within our community. Without realizing it, we are often governed by the dynamics of social identity, adopting interpretations that position us as insiders within a group and rejecting ones that position us as outsiders. The various individual "helps" and tools that are used in discipleship—daily Bible-reading notes, or Bible study guidelines—contribute to this, however well intended they may be. They reinforce the conviction that, as an evangelical for example, I ought to read this verse in a particular way. Where the need to read the Bible within the communion of the saints is acknowledged, such influence can be negotiated properly. But when we work with a basic model in which each of us reads the Bible independently, such influences become dangerous: we *assume* that a particular reading is "just what the Bible says," without recognizing and reflecting upon the extent to which we have received our interpretation from our subcultures.

Both Testaments have, as the addressees of the divine word, communities of faith. While, at points, particular messages may have come to particular figures, these were for the building up (and sometimes the tearing down) of the community, whether Israel, Judah, or the church. We will consider some of these images of community in greater depth in later chapters, but here the point that must be stressed is that this corporate dimension is basic. God's covenant with Israel may, at points, focus on an individual like David, but it is still a covenant with the nation, and his word to that people is covenantal in character. The church is the body of Christ, and its status as a community is a function of the union of each believer to Christ and thereby to every other member. None of this is intended to minimize personal responsibility or the place of personal reading of Scripture, but rather to say that each individual who reads Scripture as the word of God is already identified corporately as part of the communion of saints.

This matters because autism is a reality that is necessarily owned and faced by the community, and not just by autistic people themselves or their caregivers. The starting point for considering autism as it affects persons within the church is that it is already a reality within the body of Christ, and that the proper response to it must be made by the body. To weave this principle back into our first one: we approach autism as something that has been united to Christ and his body. Such an acknowledgment immediately highlights the problem of those who have been asked to leave churches because of difficult behaviors, and, as we will see, it will underpin the kind of attitudes that should be expected within the church.

Principle 5: We Read the Bible Humbly as a Fallible Community

It is important to our framing of the communal dimension of reading the Bible that the Scriptures we read are often directed against their readers, representing them as in dire need of correction. This is true throughout the Old Testament, and continues to be true in the New Testament. It is sobering that such criticisms and castigations are directed toward people who are nevertheless affirmed as being in Christ and filled with the Spirit. To speak of the Bible being read by the communion of saints, or the body of the church, does not make Scripture something that is owned by the church, but rather something that speaks prophetically within it.

This is important, because it prevents us from assuming that the church will automatically be a morally good, and therefore safe, environment for persons with autism or their families. Quite the opposite: we should assume that the church will be the battleground of good and evil and that those who come into the church can expect to see both lovely and ugly values at work.

To press this further, it also means that we should expect our experience of autism to expose some of those values, and to incur an obligation that we reconsider them. An important element of this involves the recognition that much of what is represented as vicious within the people of God in the Bible—what is linked to the constitutional corruption of their "flesh"—involves religious thought and practice. Throughout the Bible, the people of God (and not just those *outside* that people) are castigated for thinking wrongly about God and how they should act. This criticism is leveled as sharply at Spirit-filled people in the New Testament church as it is at those living under the old covenant; it is leveled at those who think the performance of evangelical identity necessarily involves doing a certain set of things as much as it is leveled at those who make a golden calf or commit adultery. In the case of Paul's writings, what is most striking is that he sees the problem as running so deep that those who need to be castigated are convinced within themselves that they are being faithful.

Crucially, such criticisms are leveled at people who possess the word of God and define themselves by their commitment to it. That comment may shock some readers, but it is important to recognize the truth behind it. The Pharisees, for example, were basically a renewal movement: they read their Bibles literally and called for their fellow Jews to renew their commitments to the divine commandments, to living in purity, to standing out from the wider immorality and impurity of the world—all so that they would see blessing restored to the people of God. But Jesus represented them as "children of hell" (cf. Matt 23:15) and their purity to be that of a "whitewashed tomb" (Matt 23:27).

Many of the things we consider to be good or necessary expressions of Christian thought and practice are actually products of our evangelical culture. In some cases, these may not be problematic until they are elevated into the position of idols, functioning as surrogates for the real presence of God, which disturbs and disrupts even as it enriches. Like all such surrogates, they are incapable of genuinely generating love and life and end up enslaving us to violence. They will never meet the distinctive needs of those affected by autism any more than they will meet our own needs truly; but the presence of those with autism may call attention to their emptiness and awfulness. Provided, that is, we are humble enough to exercise repentance.[26]

Where churches have asked families affected by autism not to attend because their behavior compromises the performance of the worship service, something is functioning as an idol. Where Christians undervalue others because they do not fit a certain expectation of what a believer will look and sound like, something is functioning as an idol.

Principle 6: We Read the Bible with the Spirit Who Illumines

If we are so sinful, even when we hold the word of God, how can we ever be led to truth? The answer for the New Testament writers, developed most fully (though not exclusively) by John and by Paul, is that the Holy Spirit dwells within us. He unites us to Jesus Christ, who is made actually present within us and whose mind we come to have (1 Cor 2:14). This effect of the Spirit is not represented as an instantaneous transformation that definitively eradicates sin within the church or individual Christian. Rather, we are transformed by the renewing of our mind (Rom 12:2) as the Spirit wars with our flesh (Gal 5:16-17). This is why, as I have noted above, the church must be seen as the battleground, and we must expect to encounter sin within it, even at the level of its structures.

Reading "Spiritually" most obviously entails reading prayerfully, but in a way that acknowledges particularly our need for illumination, and our instinctive preference to remain in darkness.

It is striking that one of the lengthiest expositions of the Spirit's ministry in the New Testament—Romans 8—centers on the experience of prayer by those who are beset by the world and continue to live within the limits of their sinful flesh. It is structurally important that this account is preceded by the description in Romans 7 of Paul's struggling with the continuing presence of sin in his life.[27] The representation of prayer in Romans 8 suggests that the believer's life is not one of easy triumph and success, but one of struggle and weakness. When that prayerfulness is brought to the reading of Scripture, it is powerfully liberating.

Reading Spiritually also means reading in community. Just as we can privatize our relationship with the Bible, so we can think of the Spirit as something that illuminates us individually. Consistently, though, the Spirit is represented as someone who indwells us collectively, even if that collective residing necessarily devolves to the level of the individual. His collective indwelling of us generates the unity of the church:

> For in the one Spirit we were all baptized into one body—Jews or Greeks, slaves or free—and we were all made to drink of one Spirit. (1 Cor 12:13)

The giving of the Spirit to each of us, moreover, is represented as being "for the common good" (1 Cor 12:7). This imagery is used in the context of the depiction of the church as the body of Christ, and points to the idea that the Spirit's edificational ministry is realized through the interaction of the various members, just as the flourishing of a body is realized through its parts working well together. Dynamically, this involves the kind of exchange that is represented in Colossians 3:16, interestingly also rendered in terms of indwelling.

> Let the word of Christ dwell in you richly; teach and admonish one another in all wisdom; and with gratitude in your hearts sing psalms, hymns, and spiritual songs to God.

This verse also leads us to the last point, which closes the loop with the first of our principles. The word is identified with Christ, with the language of singing psalms suggestive of the fact that the Old Testament continues to be prominently in view. And this word dwells within the body of Christ: the Spirit's indwelling work does not reidentify the body in a way that is separable from the identity of Christ, but rather realizes its identification with him. What this verse calls us to is a thoroughgoing expression of Christian identity: living in the body of Christ and allowing his voice to speak richly among us, as we speak to each other (sometimes correctively) about what is written in the whole of his word, in the Old and New Testaments.

The point is an important one because, as with the other distortions we have noted, we can consider the Spirit-filled community to be a place of victory and triumph. We can think about the Spirit in terms that are primarily about power. But he is "the Spirit of the Son" (Gal 4:6),[28] and we should expect him to manifest the Son's identity in ways that are consistent with the gospel story itself. We should expect him to be present in the kind of victory over sin that is cruciform,[29] that looks weak and fragile and unimpressive.[30] This is precisely how Paul describes the life of the church in 2 Corinthians 4, where he describes us as having "treasure in clay jars." It is not simply that these bodies are ugly shells for the indwelling glorious Spirit, but that they are vessels that continue to carry the death of Jesus within their own constitution, as a necessary part of their participation in his life (2 Cor 4:10). Within a community marked by that kind of Spirituality, the needs of those with autism, and the blessings that they can bring with their presence, can be met and realized.

Conclusions

In this chapter, I have sought to establish an interpretive framework in which we can read the Bible constructively with a view to "thinking biblically" about autism. The principles that I have laid out are not specific to an autism-oriented reading of the Bible, but bear on all interpretation of Scripture. To a significant extent, they simply reflect the "rule of faith" that governed the interpretive practices of the early church. The distinctive challenges posed by autism, however, bring the need for such principles to be observed into the foreground. If these principles are not observed or recognized, any attempt to read the Bible in relation to autism will be unsuccessful, or even counterproductive.

What the reassertion of the principles in relation to autism highlights is that a serious effort to think properly about autism brings with it a body of further blessings for the church. If we learn to think better about autism, we will learn to think better about everything else, too. And, as we will see in the next chapter, "thinking better" is something that may involve an affirmation of the cognitive and social differences in autistic people.

At the same time, if we affirm the place of those with autism in the church that is addressed by Scripture, then we also identify them as addressees. This is not an insignificant observation, for it acknowledges that the expectation of repentance and change bears upon those with autism even as it bears on others. It is all too easy to use a diagnosis of autism as an excuse to inhabit particular patterns of behavior, as a justification for actions that are hurtful to others. As we will see in chapters 3 and 4, autistic people can learn to adapt to the expectations of others and this can help them, and those around them, to flourish. As with much in this book, the application of such truths will vary according to the individual and to the specific character of their autism; the capacity for change will vary from person to person. Always, of course, the question needs to be asked: who or what ought to change, the autistic person or the neurotypical, or the world that they have made to suit them?

3

✻

AUTISM AND THE BODY OF CHRIST
Incarnation for the Church

In the preceding chapter, we identified a set of principles for how the Bible should be read in relation to autism. These principles ought to bear on all reading of the Bible, but they are pivotal to the right application of Scripture to an issue like autism. In this chapter, we will seek to implement them as we move toward a more responsible understanding of how autism should be considered in relation to the life of the church.[1]

The proposals developed in this chapter are constrained by one of the key principles that we highlighted in chapter 2: the Christian reading of Scripture must be informed and determined by the personal identity of Jesus Christ, by the mystery revealed to the saints, and by the narrative that shapes our knowledge of this identity. We worship a God who continues to bear the marks of crucifixion in the flesh that he has made to belong within his eternal life; we know him to be crucified, resurrected, and ascended, and we identify his glory with the story of his humiliation. We read New Testament authors who are insistent that this truth bore upon creation long before the temporal reality of the incarnation took place and will bear upon the future state of the creation and all who inhabit it. These authors recognize that the same single God who made all things—who bound himself in promise to Abraham, Sarah, and their descendants—is the one who is identified not just *with* but *in* Jesus. And they recognize that the identification of the one God with the cross of Jesus Christ makes no sense to the standard values of human wisdom. All of this drives them back to reconsider some of the core elements of God's dealings with the world, with insights that the authors of older Scriptures could not have been expected to enjoy.

What I want to highlight in this chapter is that the New Testament writers consistently represent God's ascription of worth and value to be different in kind from human practices. They do so, moreover in ways that intentionally *but distinctively* draw upon the representation of God in the Old Testament / Hebrew Bible. The God of Israel, incarnate in Jesus Christ, is disdainful of the kinds of social or symbolic capital that we consider to be so important, and always has been: he draws near to those whom we naturally consider to be marginal or even contemptible and elects them to involvement in his work of salvation. In his hands, those who are naturally considered worthless can be potent agents of blessing. This has an immediate bearing on how we value those with autism within the church, for God expects the same values exemplified in his work of salvation to be embodied in all those united to Christ. Persons with autism are often treated with a form of contempt within the church, just as they are in wider society. Those whose autism is less severe—who might have been diagnosed with Asperger syndrome until its removal from the diagnostic categories—are often dismissed as eccentric or are simply undervalued because they are less charismatic or "likable" than others. They may be marginalized, may be the objects of jokes, or may be seen as oddities. They do not conform to expectations; they do not fit in. Those with profound autism, meanwhile, will often exhibit disruptive behaviors that may well lead to exclusion, both for them and for their families.[2] Churches and church leaders will often pray that their numbers will grow by God providing young families, and that their needs will be met by God providing wage earners and promising future leaders; they pray, in other words, for normal solutions to the challenges they face and expect divine blessings to have such normality. The presence of a socially challenged adult with a recent diagnosis of Asperger syndrome or of a disruptive child with profound autism will not necessarily be seen as an answer to such prayers.

The values at work in the gospel challenge such perceptions of autism within the church, but they do not automatically displace them. The church cannot be assumed to constitute a safe and redemptive space for those with autism. It is the place in which the values of God's Spirit and the values of the flesh are brought into conflict, embodying a reality that continues to manifest the problems of sin. This chapter will focus on these core issues of value and the war through which they are realized within the Christian community; the next chapter will turn to some of the practical matters of how our godly evaluation of those with autism bears on our practices of accommodating their needs within the sensory and social space of the church.[3]

It is important to stress from the outset that the principles outlined in this chapter bear on how every person in the church is to be valued and on how every person in the church evaluates all others. There is a danger that a chapter such as this will be read simply as an attempt to present a condition typically seen as problematic in positive or sympathetic terms. This is not what I seek to do. Instead, I highlight that the real problem for the church is constituted by the natural evaluative intuitions by which we all ascribe worth, and that this affects attitudes toward autism in specific ways. The gospel holds this to account, but does so as it holds *all* of our judgments to account. Our reflections on autism serve to expose the presence of a wider and deeper problem.

The Incarnational Narrative and the Fourfold Gospel

When we begin to read the New Testament, within the canon of Scripture as a whole, we are first confronted with the story of Jesus of Nazareth. Two things are striking about the way that this story is told. First, it is located at its opening point—the genealogy with which Matthew begins (Matt 1:1-17)—in relation to the story of God's prior dealings with the world and particularly with the people of Israel. Second, the story is told in a fourfold form: it is recounted in the Gospels of Matthew, Mark, Luke, and John, rather than in one harmonized account. Modern biblical scholarship tends to deal with the Gospels separately, while much popular interpretation of the Gospels either replicates this separation or collapses the four into a single story, with differences flattened or explained. Theologically, neither is appropriate, for it is important that the church considered the gospel to be necessarily fourfold, allowing the differences to stand, while also refusing to allow them to split the Gospels apart. Each tells its story distinctively; each speaks to the interpretation of the other.

For this reason, we can allow the term "incarnational" to govern our readings of all four Gospels, despite the fact that this word reflects John's particular representation of Jesus as the enfleshed (i.e., in-carnate) Word. Those who read Matthew, Mark, or Luke *canonically* feel no anxiety about whether the Christology of the Synoptics involves elements that did not originally signify that Jesus was recognized to be God:[4] John's explicit identification of Jesus as the Word that became flesh informs the reading of all parts of the fourfold gospel. Biblical scholars who see their work principally as a form of historical research may want to debate the development of christological beliefs, but the theological discussion is always properly controlled by the identification of the gospel as fourfold. No distinction can be made between the "historical Jesus" and the "Christ of faith."[5]

The recognition that the fourfold gospel begins by binding the story of Jesus, through his genealogy, to the story of Israel and her Scriptures is important. It affirms these as participating in the same redemptive work of God that centers on the good news of Jesus Christ. David Bauer notes that it is formally unusual to introduce — or entitle — a genealogy with the identity of the descendant (Jesus, named in Matt 1:1), rather than the forefather (Abraham):

> The unusual practice of entitling a genealogy according to the name of the last descendant serves to subordinate the forefathers to this last descendent and indicates that they gain their meaning and identity from the final progeny, i.e., from Christ.[6]

Bauer also notes other formally surprising elements that are found in the genealogy. At key points, Matthew interrupts the normal flow of naming fathers and sons to mention two sets of brothers (the brothers of Joseph, in 1:2, and the brothers of Jechoniah at the time of the exile to Babylon, in 1:11) and to mention several women (Tamar, Rahab, Ruth, and Bathsheba, in 1:3, 1:5, and 1:6; Mary may also be included in the genealogy, in 1:17).

The mention of the brothers of Joseph, who were the fathers of the tribes of Israel (cf. Gen 46:8-25), immediately locates the story of Jesus in relation to the story of God's dealings with that people. The Word became flesh, but the particular flesh that he became was the offspring of a family whose history was defined by its special relationship to God. The mention of the brothers at the time of the exile (1:11) may be intended simply to invoke another of the major points in the history of God's dealings with this family, but it also locates what might appear to be a relationship-ending event within the lineage of God's appointed Savior: the exile, brought about in part by the persistent sins of the people, is not the end of the story of Israel's relationship with God. One important corollary of this is that the Scriptures associated with Israel continue to be associated with the redemptive work now realized in the person named Immanuel, God with Us (1:23). This is reflected in the widespread quotation of Scriptures throughout the opening chapters of Matthew. I stress this because some approaches to the theological appropriation of the New Testament break its relationship to the Old Testament / Hebrew Bible,[7] almost to the point of being functionally Marcionite. One of the regrettable results of this is that the rich material of the Old Testament that must speak to our theology—including, notably, the wisdom literature and the Psalms—is bracketed out of the theological conversation that ensues. For disability theology, in particular, this is disastrous.[8] If any given New Testament writing is set within its canonical context, though, and approached through Matthew 1, as the gateway to the wider New Testament, such an approach can be seen to be problematic.

The significance of the named women is debated and may, in fact, be polyvalent.[9] Aside from the fact that they are women,[10] they are all non-Israelites, and several have stories involving sinful elements or practices: Tamar's relationship with Judah (Gen 38) is a complicated story of sexual politics, Rahab is a prostitute, and Bathsheba (named as "the wife of Uriah," a Hittite, and thus triply identified as adulterer, foreigner, and wife to a murdered husband) slept with David while married to another man. We could, of course, dig deeper into the gendered dynamics of the stories and consider whether or to what extent the women are represented as being at fault for their sins, or whether the narration represents the male figures in each story as the true culprits and the women as sexual victims. For our purposes, the straightforward point is simply that God incorporates into his work of salvation foreigners whose lives are compromised in complicated ways by the reality of sin. They may be victims or they may be complicit, but, along with the brothers who were exiled because of their nation's sins, they are graciously involved by God in his activity to bring about redemption, to the extent of being incorporated into the very gene line of Jesus.

The mention of these women is interesting because it opens the New Testament with a particularly suggestive pattern: God involves those whom society would marginalize or treat with contempt (or even fear)—immigrants, prostitutes, adulterers, and widows—in the very lineage of the Savior. Such persons do not merely have minor cameos in the biblical material, but are pivotal to the story of God's work. We ought to expect that the New Testament church, which traces its own family history back through this one, would also be marked by such a concern to see the marginal "incorporated," that is, made part of the body; the implications for autism should be obvious.

The fourfold gospel that opens in this way continues to give us various windows onto God's care for the marginal, whether these are peripheralized by communities of faith or by society more widely. Jesus was "a friend of tax-collectors and sinners" (Matt 11:19; Luke 7:34), who made himself present with those whom many religious figures within his own community regarded as sources of contamination. He also treats with particular dignity those who were deemed of lesser value in society more generally, notably infants (Mark 10:13-15 and parallels), women (Mark 14:3-9 and parallels; John 12:1-8), and the disabled (see the cluster of stories in Matt 8–9).[11] The latter include those who are of no economic utility yet are owned and carried by their wider Jewish community, such as the paralyzed man of Matthew 9:2-8, as well as those whose conditions make them truly outsiders, such as the leper of Matthew 8:1-4, whose condition of uncleanness excluded him from the life of his religious community.

Jesus' teaching on divine providence (Matt 6:25-33 and Luke 12:22-31) connects with these stories in important ways that suggest his actions and attitudes toward the marginal are manifestations of God's own providential care for his creation. The connections are easily overlooked and need a little explanation. The parallel passages in Matthew and Luke address the anxieties that are often felt about how one (or one's family) is to be fed and clothed. In the context of the economic upheavals taking place in Galilee at the time,[12] this was probably for many people a matter of basic survival. The passages seem to indicate, though, that for others this is wrapped up with matters of status: the gentiles/nations "strive for all these things" (Matt 6:32). The aspirational language suggests that for some the anxiety might be about the *kind* of clothes worn and the *kind* of food eaten.[13] They like to eat well and dress well, something that would probably have been a visible matter of status in Galilean cities like Sepphoris and Tiberius, which were marked by the presence of both wealth and poverty. This would make sense of the location of Jesus' teaching on providence within its contexts, which, in both Matthew and Luke, concern the pursuit of status (or honor) through social, economic, and religious practices. What should, therefore, strike us when Jesus invokes God's providential care for birds and plants is that he does not focus on God's care for productive harvests, and does not use the example of doves or lambs, which could be used in religious worship. His examples involve things with no utility or value (grass and lilies) and things that would be considered unclean (ravens), and he indicates that God cares for and clothes these things in ways that exceed any human ascription of worth.[14]

We need to be careful how we draw upon these stories to frame our own moral theology or ethics. It is easy to describe Jesus as an exemplar of inclusivity, modeling life within a "brokerless kingdom,"[15] and dangerously easy to set these values against those of the Judaism of the day,[16] but he still proclaims a rigorous set of moral expectations and can speak and act in ways that seem to maintain the distinctions between God's people and outsiders.[17] He is not, in other words, quite as inclusive as we often assume.[18] We also need to be careful not to limit our values to those demonstrated *by* Jesus at the expense of other New Testament passages that speak of values as manifested by the community *in* him. This is to recognize that the moral vision of the New Testament is not simply one of following Jesus, but one of living in him, of sharing in his eschatological life and identity through the activity of the Holy Spirit.[19] The approach that asks "What would Jesus do?" limits its moral resources in unhelpful ways that end up being mere exemplarism. What the New Testament leads us toward is something more radical, which involves our participation in Christ and the work of the Spirit in making that participation a reality in our lives. The fourfold incarnational narrative remains the central description of the identity of Jesus, but it is placed within theological accounts of the wider New Testament and within the canon as a whole; it does not stand alone.

The Gospel narratives culminate with the accounts of crucifixion and resurrection, followed in Luke with the description of the ascension. It is, of course, highly suggestive for theologies of both disability and trauma that Jesus is maimed and disfigured in his mortality and that this is redemptively significant. John's Gospel, in fact, seems to identify the sufferings of Christ with his glory, in ways that are subversive and suggestive at once (notably in John 12:23, but arguably also in 3:14, 8:28, and 12:32). It makes no earthly sense, but the sufferings of Jesus constitute

God's triumph over evil. This element is picked up in the wider New Testament, both as the basis for a radical reevaluation of human standards of worth and as a new framework within which to understand human suffering.

While the gospel narratives culminate with these events, however, they do not effectively *finish* there. Luke continues his account with the book of Acts, narrating the continuing work of Christ and his Spirit through the church as it begins to grow and spread outward from Jerusalem and through the wider Roman world. Canonically, this book (much of which is taken up with the story of the apostle Paul) follows the Gospels and forms a bridge between them and the Epistles. Three things might be noted as especially significant. First, the church is identified with the continuing life of the risen and ascended Jesus: when Saul (Paul) is confronted by the risen Christ, the latter asks, "Saul, Saul, why do you persecute *me*?" (Acts 9:4). This is to say that Christ is present in the suffering of his church. Second, as the church that participates in his life, the community of believers is characterized by God's incarnational care for the needy and marginal, practicing a community of goods that is not only charitable, but also entails a sacrificing of status and stratification (Acts 4:32-37). Third, as this church grows, God adds to its number by incorporating gentiles into the community of Christ, transcending (if not effacing) the boundaries and distinctions between Israel and the world, between clean and unclean.

The very core of the gospel story involves a recognition that God loves the unlovely, the things that are generally considered difficult to love and that are typically treated with contempt, and makes them pivotal to a work of salvation that itself centers on a moment of extreme unloveliness. God chooses immigrants and sinners to carry forward the genetic material of the one who will die as a criminal, so that the marginal can be made central to the community of salvation. This is not just about his love for sinners, but about his whole attitude toward the creation, which is populated by the clean and the unclean, the pretty and the grotesque, the sparrows and the ravens. Those united to the life of this God through the gospel are expected to manifest the same values, refusing to ascribe worth on the basis of perceived capital and instead showing love and care to those who would naturally be treated with scorn, fear, or loathing.

This is profoundly important to the question of how we consider autism. Most people tend to value normality, to be drawn to beauty and to value things with obvious capital value. They like the "likable," who are like themselves. They value those who demonstrate their worth by participating in the social world and performing well; they ascribe particular value to those who outperform others. Whether it is recognized or not, the ascription of value is competitive—some win and some lose—and the rules of the competition are generally social and economic. Those with autism are likely to be considered of less value when people think in these ways: they are not *always* easy to like, they do not *always* bring much social capital, they may have little utilitarian value to the community. But believers have been united through Christ to the one who loves the ravens and incorporates immigrants into the genealogy of Jesus; they have a responsibility to see all fellow members as objects of God's providence and as vitally part of his church. Once they do so, they can begin to comprehend the part that those who do not fit the pattern of "normality" might play in the organism that is the body of Christ.

The True Image of God

The perceived continuity of the gospel with the story of Israel led early Christians, including the New Testament writers, to read the Old Testament in new ways that were shaped by their conviction that the identity of Jesus Christ, disclosed in the incarnational narrative, is the mystery that makes sense of everything. They made figural connections between Jesus and persons or concepts in the Old Testament that appeared to have their own discrete identity, but that were now understood differently in the light of Christ.

Perhaps the most important example of this is the "image of God." The new incarnational understanding of this has profound implications for the way we think about autism. In Genesis 1:26-27, humanity is described as created "in" (or "according to") the "image" and "likeness" of God. It is important that the language of Genesis controls the significance of the image/likeness through the use of prepositions: humans are "in" (Hebrew: *bᵉ*) or "according to/after" (Greek: *kata*) the image. This prevents us from seeing humans *as* the image. In fact, some Jewish readings understand the relationship between the words "image" and "likeness" as a genitive chain, so that humanity is "in the image of the likeness," something that ensures even greater distinction between humans and the image.[20] By contrast, the New Testament writers consider that Jesus, the object of their worship and allegiance, *is* the image (Col 1:15; 2 Cor 4:4). For Paul, this means that Jesus is the legitimate *icon* through whom we can worship the one God properly, something that ties in strongly with his concern to maintain proper monotheism against idolatry and is closely connected to the way that he represents Jesus as the visible glory of God.[21] Jesus and Jesus alone is the image in this sense; the image-bearing of other humans is derivative—they are patterned "after" the image.[22]

This may not sound immediately relevant to autism, but it is profoundly important because it represents all human image-bearing as participatory. The true image cannot be identified with a particular set of characteristics, capacities, or properties enjoyed by all complete human beings, the absence of which compromises that image. Such a way of thinking about the *imago Dei* can be observed at various points in the Christian tradition, but can result in a view of disability that sees the individuals who lack certain abilities or properties as constituting "defective" images of God.[23] Now, we might acknowledge that we all bear the image of God defectively, in some sense, because of our sinfulness, but this way of thinking moves further and sees something fundamentally lacking in the disabled person: they fall short of being a real image of God because of their impairment. A corollary of this is the expectation that this deficiency will be fixed when we are raised to eternal life, which is an issue that we will discuss further in the conclusion. By contrast, a participatory account of the image, which understands human image-bearing to derive its significance from the nonsubstitutable identity of Jesus,[24] avoids the notion that the elements of the image can be identified with a particular combination of properties, considered on their own terms. Instead, all who have a kinship with Jesus through their common human nature share in his image-bearing, and those united to him by his Spirit are transformed into the likeness of that image in a distinctive and dynamic way (2 Cor 3:18).[25]

This way of thinking about the image may sound strange to us, but it is a standard concept in the early patristic material, as the fathers of the church read the New Testament and seek to develop an account of salvation that does justice to the way the biblical authors represent the gospel. The fathers are concerned to articulate this in a way that takes seriously and integrates three striking elements of the biblical teaching: (1) the significance of the incarnation predates the life of Jesus and even the existence of the cosmos (Col 1:15-23; John 1:1-4), meaning that (2) all things are "in Christ" in some sense and humans are image-bearers in a special way (Col 1:17), while (3) there is a distinctive sense in which those who believe, who are filled with the Spirit and who partake of the sacraments, are "in Christ" and share in his image (2 Cor 3:18). The fathers make careful and judicious use of Platonic categories of nature, which allow them to see things that share a nature as participating in a common reality: two dogs may be quite different in shape and character, suffering various degrees of imperfection, but they share a nature and hence participate in something that unifies them, what we might call their common "dogness." The same kinship binds humans, who share a human nature. The fathers consider it vital that Jesus shares in our humanity and that his uniting of this to the eternal and unchanging life of God is key, not only to salvation, but to all of God's dealings with the world. They were not, in any simple sense, Platonists, but these categories of *nature* and *being* allowed them to see our natural human kinship with Jesus as making possible a participation in the life of God himself. The principle can be traced widely in the patristic writings throughout the early centuries of the church and across its geographical spread,[26] but it is especially well developed in Athanasius' sustained reflection *On the Incarnation*.[27] One particular passage is worth quoting at length, for reasons that will quickly become evident:

> Thus, because he envies nothing its existence, he made everything from nothing through his own Word, our Lord Jesus Christ. And among these creatures, of all those on earth he had special pity for the human race, and seeing that by the definition of its own existence it would be unable to persist forever, he gave it an added grace, not simply creating men like all irrational animals on the earth, but making them in his own image and giving them also *a share* in the power of his own Word, so that *having as it were shadows of the Word* and being made rational, they might be able to remain in felicity and live the true life in paradise, which is really that of the saints.[28]

This is a description of the creation of humanity, and precedes his discussion of the fall. What is most important to note is that Athanasius represents human image-bearing as involving analogy or correspondence (humans have "shadows of the Word") and a "share" of participation in the "rational" Word, the mind of God. The kinship between us and the image is rendered, then, particularly in terms of reason, but in a way that assumes that all human participation in this is partial. However impaired, deficient, or simply different the reason or rationality of a person may be, they still have "shadows" and a "share" of the Word that was made flesh. The key point of note is precisely that the capacity to accommodate varying degrees of a property within human image-bearing reflects its participatory and derivative character.[29]

Again, the relevance of this to autism should be obvious. The image of God is often conceived in ways that tie it to certain capacities, configured in a typical way. If the participatory character of Athanasius' account is not grasped, his own emphasis on rationality would appear to make the image something that is particularly associated with typical cognitive ability. Others have seen the image as a social reality, embodied in our capacity to enjoy relationships with other people and with God. Those who are autistic, whose cognitive development is different (at best) and may be severely affected by their condition, can be seen as defective versions of the image and placed in a category apart from other humans. Their difficulties with social experience can be seen as a more fundamental defect, compromising even further the possibility that they can be identified with the image of God. In some theological approaches, in fact, the "defects" of autism are used to cast light on the "normal" social function that is taken for granted, with the labels "autism" and "autist" coming to function with essentially pejorative significance, even if applied in symbolic ways: those who fall short of true fellowship with God are "spiritual autists." I consider this mode of reflection on autism to be problematic. Recovering the participatory theology of the *imago Dei* that marked the fathers, which is not identical to the accounts of the image that developed in later traditions, might be a helpful counter to this.

The Scandal of the Cross and the Absurdity of Election

When Paul writes to the church in Corinth, he challenges a range of behaviors and attitudes that he considers to be incompatible with life in Christ, the image of God, into whose likeness we are metamorphosing.[30] The Corinthians evince values that appear to be little different from those of the society around them, particularly as they ascribe honor and practice religion. They are, for the most part (and I choose this word carefully), perfectly "normal" in the way that they think and act: they are impressed by smart people and powerful teachers; they treat the wealthy as more important than the poor; they see some as more valuable to the church than others, because of their gifts and abilities or their capital resources. These were values that Corinthians would consider quite appropriate, even as we do today, even if some of us do not like to admit it. But Paul challenges them, because these entirely normal values have now been exposed by the gospel to reflect our constitutional sinfulness, our natural opposition to God's value system.

Paul's word for this constitutional sinfulness is "flesh" (*sarx*), and it important to appreciate how he now understands it in relation to the gospel. In his second letter to the Corinthians, he writes:

> [16] From now on, therefore, we regard no one from a human point of view (lit.: according to the flesh, *kata sarka*); even though we once knew Christ from a human point of view (*kata sarka*), we know him no longer in that way. [17] So if anyone is in Christ, there is a new creation: everything old has passed away; see, everything has become new! (2 Cor 5:16-17)

Much has been written on Paul's use of "flesh" as an expression for the sinful nature,[31] but it most naturally indicates that sin is not simply something that we do, but something that inheres in our being. Crucially, this thing distorts our values and affects our ability to perceive truth; we understand the world sinfully, "according to the flesh," *kata sarka*. Paul's encounter with Christ and consequent union with him, by which he is "in Christ," disrupts this reality. Everything has become new, and Paul no longer knows Christ "according to the flesh"; now he knows Christ according to what was revealed to him.

This has a profound effect on Paul's understanding of the values that necessarily accompany the gospel and how these bear on his previous way of thinking about value. Where he previously attached capital significance to various things that were true of him—as in Philippians 3:4-6, where he talks about his family background and his performance of Jewish identity—now he recognizes that this symbolic capital is worthless and fouled.[32] The things that he used to see as impressive and important, and that he assumed would be impressive to God as well as to other people, he now sees for what they truly are. And he expects other Christians to do the same.

When this is brought back to 1 Corinthians 1, it casts interesting light on the dynamics at work in the texts. Paul begins by condemning the fact that there are factions in Corinth that have grown up around particular figures:

> Each of you says, "I belong to Paul," or "I belong to Apollos," or "I belong to Cephas," or "I belong to Christ." (1 Cor 1:12)

There is no reason to think that these figures have invited such support (the presence of both Paul and Christ on the list would tell against this), but it is natural and normal for people to form such groups, whether invited to or not. Paul challenges the basic factionalism by pointing to the unity of the body of Christ ("Has Christ been divided?" 1 Cor 1:13), and this theme continues to run through the epistle. He also digs deeper, though, into the kinds of values that underpin the formation of these groups and the other divisions that mark the Corinthian church, as members are separated into groups of different social value. This is where his language of "flesh" as a value-distorting constitutional problem comes into play.

He begins by indicating that the message of the cross does not conform to human wisdom, and he calls into question the value systems with which that wisdom operates:

> [18] For the message about the cross is foolishness to those who are perishing, but to us who are being saved it is the power of God. [19] For it is written,
>
>> "I will destroy the wisdom of the wise,
>> and the discernment of the discerning I will thwart."
>
> [20] Where is the one who is wise? Where is the scribe? Where is the debater of this age? Has not God made foolish the wisdom of the world? [21] For since, in the wisdom of God, the world did not know God through wisdom, God decided, through the foolishness of our proclamation, to save those who believe. (1 Cor 1:18-21)

The use of the connective "for" (*gar*) at the beginning of this statement links it to the discussion that has gone before, which concerns the existence of factions within the church. Those factions probably came into being because of the natural or intuitive tendency to ascribe worth to people who are considered to be impressive. Ancient literature reflects an awareness that this is not just a matter of intelligence, but of "presence": philosophers would learn to speak with deep voices and to stand with impressive postures, even shaving their limbs for effect, in order to be perceived as figures of strength. This could also be wrapped up in the dynamics of "patronage," both at the formal level of an actual patron-client relationship, where someone has a wealthy sponsor, and at a less formal level of opinion: if a person of standing is particularly well inclined toward a particular teacher, that will carry weight with certain people.

The dynamic we have described is not dissimilar to the one that gives rise to groups within contemporary Christianity that are particularly identified with certain prominent Bible teachers, who are usually distinguished by being excellent communicators and skilled orators; they speak well, and people warm to that. This is a particularly visible form of the general tendency to ascribe value to all people who are socially impressive in some way. These are the people the church celebrates, and its structures and practices are often built around this celebration: significant space is typically carved out for the delivery of an act of oratory, framed by music led by charismatic performers, followed by social times in which we can enact our precious normality. My intention here is not to sound cynical or dismissive of these things, which can be valuable and helpful, but to recognize that they can also easily become vehicles for our natural tendencies to respond intuitively to the socially impressive qualities of others, or even to warm to their sheer normality. Those same things can be contexts in which contempt for the non-normal can be displayed: while the celebrity preacher speaks, the person with profound autism may be acting disruptively, much to the chagrin of others; during the social time afterwards, the person with autism may be physically marginal (standing in a corner) or may even have left because of social distress. While most in the congregation respond positively to the preacher's message, delivered with such panache, the person with autism may be unaffected by the rhetoric and see straight through to the points of misconception that underlie it; when they share this perception with others, they can be seen as arrogant or unspiritual. When leadership elections come around, no one considers the person with autism as a candidate, because autism is often not easily "likable."

Those with autism frequently lack the kinds of impressive qualities or charisma that cause people to "like" others and to value them as members of the community. Even within the church, we like people to be funny, clever, and socially competent: we are drawn to those qualities, and consider the people who embody them to be important parts of our church. If they were to leave our fellowship, we would feel that we had lost something important. If there is a need for leadership, these are the people whom we feel ought to be in the role. Those with autism, though, do not always elicit a similar response. There are funny, clever, and socially competent people with autism (though the social dimension may be exhausting for them), but there are also many with autism who have no such social capital. But God chose "the things that are not, to reduce to nothing the things that are" (1 Cor 1:28): if we value people less because they lack the qualities that are socially impressive, we are a long way from embodying God's love. Again, I do not intend for this to sound cynical or sweeping; there are many churches, and many people throughout the worldwide church, of which or of whom this could not be said. We need to be aware, though, that these subtle dynamics are at work all the time, and that any of us may participate in such values, even without recognizing it.

But the message of the cross cannot be accommodated within this. There is no way to make a crucified criminal, forced to suffer a shameful death, socially impressive. If the gospel proclamation centers on such an event, the life of those saved through this gospel cannot continue to be governed by the values of earthly wisdom, which see wealth and strength and honor as the key goods. Paul goes on to describe "Christ crucified" as a "stumbling block to Jews and foolishness to Gentiles" (1 Cor 1:23); to those who are "the called" (*tois klētois*), however, this same figure is "the power of God and the wisdom of God" (1 Cor 1:24). These are interesting designations, for while they may connote certain Old Testament passages, they also represent a dramatic subversion of the categories of honor: this crucified man is now the true emblem of wisdom and the true emblem of might, and our thinking must be brought in line with this.

The term "the called" (*tois klētois*) invokes the concept of election or divine choosing. Throughout the Bible, this concept is deployed in a somewhat subversive way, with God making surprising choices of whom to involve in his work. This is most strikingly true in relation to Israel:

> ⁷ It was not because you were more numerous than any other people that the LORD set his heart on you and chose you—for you were the fewest of all peoples. ⁸ It was because the Lord loved you and kept the oath that he swore to your ancestors, that the LORD has brought you out with a mighty hand, and redeemed you from the house of slavery, from the hand of Pharaoh king of Egypt. (Deut 7:7-8)

God's election of Israel is not a cause for boasting; it is, in fact, something that disdains all human standards of respect for power. Instead, it is traced to God's free decision to love Israel: he set his affection on you because he loved you.

When we continue to read in Deuteronomy, this principle of election continues to be developed and applied in interesting ways:

> ¹⁴ Although heaven and the heaven of heavens belong to the LORD your God, the earth with all that is in it, ¹⁵ yet the LORD set his heart in love on your ancestors alone and chose you, their descendants after them, out of all the peoples, as it is today. ¹⁶ Circumcise, then, the foreskin of your heart, and do not be stubborn any longer. ¹⁷ For the LORD your God is God of gods and Lord of lords, the great God, mighty and awesome, who is not partial and takes no bribe, ¹⁸ who executes justice for the orphan and the widow, and who loves the strangers, providing them food and clothing. ¹⁹ You shall also love the stranger, for you were strangers in the land of Egypt. (Deut 10:14-19)

God's sovereign choice is here disaligned with the power values of the world and directed toward those who are without
commodity or capital value: widows, orphans, immigrants. He
expects those whom he has elected to share in that value system, loving the stranger as God has loved them. We have seen
already that that the genealogy of Jesus is recounted in such a
way as to highlight the presence of widows, immigrants, and
sinners in the lineage of the Savior; Paul similarly draws upon
the biblical tradition of countercapitalistic election in his challenge to the value system of the Corinthians.

Paul expands on this reference to election in the following
verses, drawing into it the language of "flesh":

> [26] Consider your own call, brothers and sisters: not many of
> you were wise by human standards (*kata ʃarka*), not many
> were powerful, not many were of noble birth. [27] But God
> chose what is foolish in the world to shame the wise; God
> chose what is weak in the world to shame the strong; [28] God
> chose what is low and despised in the world, things that are
> not (*ta mē onta*), to reduce to nothing things that are, [29] so that
> no one might boast in the presence of God. [30] He is the source
> of your life in Christ Jesus, who became for us wisdom from
> God, and righteousness and sanctification and redemption.
> (1 Cor 1:26-30)

Paul here asserts that God's electing activity is attached to "the
things that are not" (*ta mē onta*), which he "chooses" to nullify "the
things that are" (*ta onta*). This is a radical and fundamental rejection of our natural evaluative principles, at the most basic level. It
understands God's election to be entirely disdainful of any account
of worth that is based on perceived commodity or capital: by definition, "the things that are not" are without capital of any sort, and
yet these are the things that are celebrated by God.

The same emphasis on the incongruity of God's electing
work runs through the rest of 1 Corinthians and emerges with
particular force in Paul's description of the Eucharist (1 Cor

11:17-34). The reference to all eating their own meals, with some going hungry while others get drunk (11:21), is often understood to reflect the social stratification that would have affected the dining practices of ancient feasts. Following a classic study by Jerome Murphy-O'Connor that examined the architecture of ancient ruins in Corinth,[33] the assumption has generally been made that wealthy members of the church were seated in a heated main room (*triclinium*) and ate first, while poorer members were placed in an unheated room (*atrium*) and ate only once the main group had eaten their fill. Hence, when Paul addresses those who have homes of their own in which to eat and drink, and castigates them for humiliating "those who have nothing" (*ta mē echontas*), he is challenging those who sit at the main table in the atrium and eat without care for the poorer members of the community who are seated elsewhere and out of sight. Some more recent research on less wealthy parts of the city, where houses could not afford a separate eating space for the lower classes, has suggested that this reconstruction is not necessarily correct.[34] Still, Paul's language suggests that those who go hungry are the "have nots," a suggestive translation that highlights the division of those attending Eucharist according to social status. The expression *ta mē echontas* is strikingly parallel to *ta mē onta*: "the have nots" and "the are nots" are objects of contempt when judged "according to the flesh," but they have been chosen by God to nullify the world's values.

Paul's response to this division centers on the symbolism of the Lord's Supper as a participation in the "body of the Lord":

> For all who eat and drink without discerning the body, eat and drink judgment against themselves. (1 Cor 11:29)

Contextually, "discerning the body" must be understood to designate a recognition of the shared union with Christ that binds all Christians to each other. In the previous chapter, Paul has used the imagery of body and bread with precisely this force:

> [16] The cup of blessing that we bless, is it not a sharing in the blood of Christ? The bread that we break, is it not a sharing in the body of Christ? [17] Because there is one bread, we who are many are one body, for we all partake of the one bread. (1 Cor 10:16-17)

In the following chapter, Paul expands on this identification of the church as the body of Christ. The image of a multipartite but unified body affirms the diversity of the constituent members under the controlling motif of "gift." The condition of each part of the body is "given" by the one God, who is now identified as Father, Son, and Spirit:

> [4] Now there are varieties of gifts, but the same Spirit; [5] and there are varieties of services, but the same Lord; [6] and there are varieties of activities, but it is the same God who activates all of them in everyone. [7] To each is given the manifestation of the Spirit for the common good. (1 Cor 12:4-7)

This "manifestation of the Spirit" includes the "spiritual gifts" that can be categorized and listed, but it also involves properties such as "faith" (1 Cor 12:9). Paul's description moves from these gifts to speaking in more general terms about diversity within the body:

> [12] For just as the body is one and has many members, and all the members of the body, though many, are one body, so it is with Christ. [13] For in the one Spirit we were all baptized into one body—Jews or Greeks, slaves or free—and we were all made to drink of one Spirit. (1 Cor 12:12-13)

The emphasis, then, falls on a "given" or "gifted" corporate reality, involving a union of ethnically and socially diverse individuals, with a range of natural and charismatic abilities. Their unity, importantly, is derived not from any values or properties that they naturally share as people, but rather from a common alien reality that has been given to each of them: the Holy Spirit. As I have written elsewhere:

> The membership of the body, with all its diversity, owes its presence to the work of God: each member is given *to* the body by God and is gifted *within* the body by God: Each individual, with their capacities and their burdens, their strengths and their deficits, is "owned" by the community within an economy of gift, something that cuts across the economy of capital or commodity that we have seen to be at work.[35]

This is profoundly significant for how the church thinks about persons with autism. Rather than, in the first instance, being considered to be marginal or to be burdens, people who are tolerated or accepted, but not celebrated, they are considered to be *givens*, received with joy and thanksgiving. They are gifts, as are all members of the body. Then, and only then, can the burdens and the abilities that they bring be considered and addressed, as realities owned, borne, and enjoyed by the community.

> [21] The eye cannot say to the hand, "I have no need of you," nor again the head to the feet, "I have no need of you." [22] On the contrary, the members of the body that seem to be weaker are indispensable, [23] and those members of the body that we think less honorable we clothe with greater honor, and our less respectable members are treated with greater respect; [24] whereas our more respectable members do not need this. But God has so arranged the body, giving the greater honor to the inferior member, [25] that there may be no dissension within the body, but the members may have the same care for one another. [26] If one member suffers, all suffer together with it; if one member is honored, all rejoice together with it. (1 Cor 12:21-26)

We will see in chapter 4 something of how this bears on the obligation of members of the body to accommodate the special needs of others. Here the point is simply that the value of members is not grounded in their perceived social capital, but rather on the fact that they have been chosen by God, given to the body, and gifted with the Holy Spirit, even in ways that are unremarkable. Their presence is a cause for celebration, and their suffering is a cause for collective concern. This is true of all members, and bears upon all of our values.

Paul's teaching on the Lord's Supper and on the body of Christ speaks to the way that we think about all disability, not just autism, within the church, but it does so by identifying all members of the body (not just the disabled) in terms of their union with Christ. The starting point for all reflection must be the category of "gift":[36] those who are affected by various conditions that affect the social capital that the world would ascribe to them have a value within the body of Christ that cannot be reduced to their abilities or contributions. They are valuable because they have been chosen by God and given to the body of Christ. They will enrich the community, which would in important ways be dismembered by their absence, but this cannot be judged only in terms of the contribution that we would expect them to make. It can never be reduced to utility. This is true of the person with autism, and it is true of the neurotypical.

It is important that this colors the ways that the value of those with autism is defended. It is always tempting to make such a defense on the basis of the particular strengths that those with autism might bring. Such contributions should, of course, be recognized. We can fall into the trap, however, of ascribing value to autism only insofar as it confers unique abilities. We can value the person who is brilliant at science, or math, or linguistics, or theology because of the unusual capacity to understand systems or to sustain attention that often goes with autism. The danger is that such an approach has no room to value the person who is nonverbal, profoundly affected by autism and requiring lifelong care. To see the autistic person as a gift and as a member of the body, however, ascribes to them a value that is irreducible, that transcends contributions without negating them, and that is traced back to the very love of God.

The Church as the Battleground of Flesh and Spirit

By this point, the study of 1 Corinthians should have made something glaringly obvious. The church is not a safe place just because it is the church. It is not a place where the values of God's kingdom are straightforwardly implemented and applied to the welfare of each member. It is the place where the battle of the flesh and the Spirit occurs most violently, and it may, therefore, continue to be full of dangers for its vulnerable members. They can be marginalized, disdained, hated, and mistreated by those who call upon the name of the Lord. This is wrong, but it is also the reality. Furthermore, this reality is embodied within Christian communities that wrongly perceive their viciousness to be religious virtuosity: Paul, after all, writes to a community within which a particular group of people presses for a particular set of behaviors because they are convinced that it is religiously correct to do so. He even has to challenge a fellow apostle, Peter, for being drawn into supporting this way of thinking (Gal 2:11). It is a salutary lesson, repeated throughout the New Testament and reflecting much in the prophetic writings of the Old Testament, that simply belonging to the people of God does not exempt us from the possibility that we will act viciously, with the best of religious intentions. Nothing should make us expect that churches will be safe spaces for the vulnerable; they will only become so through the Spirit's war with the flesh.

This language of warfare between the flesh and the Spirit is developed by Paul in Galatians 5:13-26, the beginning of which reads:

> [13] For you were called to freedom, brothers and sisters; only do not use your freedom as an opportunity for self-indulgence, but through love become slaves to one another. [14] For the

whole law is summed up in a single commandment, "You shall love your neighbor as yourself." [15] If, however, you bite and devour one another, take care that you are not consumed by one another.

[16] Live by the Spirit, I say, and do not gratify the desires of the flesh. [17] For what the flesh desires is opposed to the Spirit, and what the Spirit desires is opposed to the flesh; for these are opposed to each other, to prevent you from doing what you want. (Gal 5:13-17)

There are two important points to highlight here. First, Paul highlights that Christian freedom is not a warrant for self-interest, as we see ourselves freed from the obligation to act in particular ways. Rather, it is a freedom that empowers us, through love, to serve each other. The NRSV translation captures nicely the force of the verb *douleuō*: "to serve as slaves." We have been released from a tyrannical slavery to a single master, Sin, but are now called to serve each other. We are not yet freed from the reality of our embodiment within weak flesh, though, and the instinct "to bite and devour" each other continues to make itself known, with its inevitably destructive outcome: we "consume" each other (5:15). As an aside, the overtones of that word are not incidental: when our constitutional sinfulness expresses itself, it often does so in ways that assimilate the values of the church to the values of the consumer.

Second, his final statement—"so that you are not able to do what you want" (5:17, my translation)—has a force that is worth probing. It is often understood as if it merely indicates our repeated failure to obey God: our flesh wars with the Spirit and prevents us from obeying God as the Spirit seeks to lead us to do. The grammatical construction, however, suggests that the expression is better understood as "you may not (i.e., you are not allowed) to do the things that you wish."[37] That is, it is not permissible to do what we might wish; our instincts and preferences are held to account by the Spirit's present. Christian formation, then, involves a deliberate mistrust of the instincts of our flesh.

Something important needs to noted here, though with some care. These "fleshly" instincts will be different in different persons. Those with autism may, in fact, be free from some of the sinful instincts of others precisely because of their social difficulties. They may lack the kinds of instincts that lead others to intuitively ascribe worth to the socially impressive. This is one of the reasons, in fact, that autistic people are often seen to be rude or arrogant, and one of the reasons that they often refuse to be pulled into the social dynamics of churches. They lack the capacity to participate in some of the sinful value systems that compromise others. Reflecting on their difficulties with the church culture may, in fact, be an important constructive part of the church's ongoing reflections on what is wrong and sinful in its practices.

We must not be crass or naïve in this, however, and must not romanticize autism, as if those who are autistic are blissfully free of sin. We will consider some particularly severe challenges that they face in chapter 5. Here we will simply note that those with autism are confronted by the values of the gospel, even as they are affirmed by them. Those with autism participate in the war of flesh and Spirit as much as anyone else does, and autistic Christians have a responsibility (albeit one that will bear differently on each person according to their cognitive abilities) to pursue an identity defined principally by Christ and not by their autism. While this needs to be said carefully, it does need to be said: autistic people can sometimes be genuinely hurtful to those around them and can be genuinely selfish, in ways that are shaped by their neurotype. One danger with an autism diagnosis is always that it can be used as a license to remain fixed within patterns of behavior that are unloving. The potential for autistic people to adapt has already been noted, however, and we have highlighted their capacity to develop empathy and to acquire understanding of others through processes of learning and formation.[38] For autistic Christians, Paul's warning that "you may not do what you want" carries a particular force, which shows everyone their need for the Spirit to work change within them, through which they will be led into a condition of true flourishing.

Conclusion

Within the church, we often form a sense of inclusion through "normal" social practices, and those same practices influence the ways in which we ascribe relative value to other Christians. Those who are like us, who share our jargon, are good at social practices, make the right kind of eye contact, and say the right things, are the kinds of people whom we consider to be insiders and whom we value as members of our churches. Those who are particularly impressive, who are great speakers or charismatic "people persons," we see as candidates for leadership, whether at a formal level or just at the intuitive level as people worth following. Autistic people, however, often lack the ability to perform these kinds of skills effectively and are often marginalized. They may not be excluded from a church (although those with profound autism and the disruptive behavior that goes with it may well be), but they will probably be marginalized in some way. The decision to label someone as "on the spectrum" is normally a dismissive one, which functions to identify the person as someone we tolerate but would not be sad to see leave our church.

We have seen, however, that the New Testament writers draw upon the Old Testament imagery of election to render the truth that they see played out in the gospel of Jesus Christ: God chooses the things that people tend to marginalize, scorn, and even fear to participate in his work of salvation. He includes immigrants and prostitutes in the lineage of Jesus, and chooses "the things that are not" to nullify the things that the world considers important. He chooses these things and gives them as gifts to the community that he is saving in Jesus Christ. They are gifts that bring burdens, to be sure, but they are holy and special "givens" for the church and must be treated with all the care and love that we would lavish on any royal gift.

And, of course, God's work of saving such things involves an act of deliverance, a victory over the power that enslaves, won through a reality that involves shame, suffering, and exclusion. Jesus is crucified outside the city, and we must not lose sight of how senseless his death is according to the logics of the world. Our flesh will continue to war with the Spirit and will continue to invest itself in religious values entirely at odds with the gospel, even in our account of the gospel itself. But the Spirit holds those values to account, and those with autism may play an important part in the church's ongoing repentance over values that do not serve the objects of God's election in love and kindness.

4

AUTISM IN THE CHURCH
A Sensory Space for All God's People

Autistic people have neurological characteristics that mean they experience social interaction and the sensory world differently than the wider population. Interactions that others would find easy, spontaneous, and energizing may for them be difficult, studied, and exhausting; nonverbal communicative acts that others would find clear may for them be opaque. The subtext to a conversation, or the unstraightforward use of language, may be difficult to comprehend. The sights, sounds, smells, tastes, and touches that attend these interactions may be distracting or overwhelming for some, while for others they may not even register. In the case of profoundly autistic persons, challenging or even disturbing behaviors may take the place of normal participation in this environment. If such social and sensory challenges can be difficult in day-to-day life, they are intensively so in the context of the church, in worship services awash with stimuli, set within an expectation that the church "community" will express itself in accepted ways. Badly set-up sound systems, flickering lights, loud bands, loud voices, hand soap, hair products, perfume, deodorant, breath—there is a long and varied list of stimuli that for many will be unpleasant at best and for others will be overwhelming. Services may involve some time devoted to social interaction—a time of greeting or the exchanging of peace—and will usually be preceded or followed by a more extended time of "fellowship." Such times may be uncomfortable or challenging for a person with autism, or difficult for parents of children with autism, especially when disapproval of certain behaviors may be unambiguously visible.

While these experiences have no doubt caused some with autism to give up or avoid attending church services, others continue to be involved in such gatherings. In some cases, perhaps, this is simply a matter of observing what appears to be non-negotiable expectation in the New Testament writings: Christians must not give up meeting together (Heb 10:25). In many cases, however, those with autism find participation in the fellowship of believers to be a genuine blessing, bringing friendship, support, and a valuable opportunity to join with others in praising God. We need to be careful not to reinforce stereotypes about autism by underrepresenting this particular capacity for participation.

But even those who value their participation in communities of faith will find elements of this to be difficult; or, conversely, people in the community of faith will find autistic individuals difficult. Communities involve communication, and that is something that may be problematized where there are autistic people, either because of misunderstandings or because of a clearly understood degree of honesty that is not considered socially acceptable. The results may be innocuous, or they may result in long-term damage to relationships. For pastors and fellow believers, it is vital to be aware of the kinds of experiences that might arise in such a context.

Social Bonds and Unity in the Body of Christ

As discussed in chapter 3, Paul's language of "the flesh" calls into question the ways that we tend to ascribe value through instinctive but often problematic social performances. This bears also on communal identity. Groups define their boundaries—the lines that separate the insider from the outsider—on the basis of a shared set of convictions, practices, and behaviors, the significance of which is often recognized tacitly without being questioned. Within the group, the perceived competency with which individuals perform this identity will become the basis for how they are evaluated and placed within the group's hierarchy, whether this is formalized or not. One way to describe the value that is placed on these performances is to consider them as constituting a form of "symbolic capital" or "social capital." The ascription of such capital reflects the group and its subcultural values: someone outside the group may see no value or worth in a specific person's life, where those inside may see it as evidence of their worthiness to be ascribed status. Such practices are not necessarily wrong, but they are always held to account by the gospel. They are instinctive for us, but the instincts behind them may be compromised by sin. Importantly, and functionally, the ways that we express and experience Christian unity are often determined significantly by these, and not adequately by the strategies of identity formation that are visible in the writings of the New Testament authors.

It is important to recognize that several of the New Testament authors challenge their reading communities to devote sustained attention to particular imaginative representations of Christian unity and value. These are metaphors or images that represent the church as a unity, though often in ways that highlight the internal diversity of which that unity is comprised. The most obvious example of this is the image of the church as the body of Christ, which Paul develops at length in 1 Corinthians 12 and more briefly elsewhere. Alongside this, we find the image of the church as God's temple, which is developed both by Paul and by Peter in ways that suggest the unity of the Christian community, and the image of the church as branches of a vine, which John reports in the Fourth Gospel.

Several points may be noted in relation to these images. First, each is quite concrete in character. That is, each represents the unity of the church in ways that are comprehensible to anyone who has seen a physical body, building, or plant. The relating of "oneness" or unity to diversity is accomplished through images that are straightforward to understand as depictions of single things that are made up of several parts. This is important because, for many with autism, such "concrete images" are readily grasped and are, indeed, crucial as imaginative devices for understanding complex realities. Temple Grandin, for example, speaks of constructing an imaginative picture of complex realities out of photographic memories of the various parts of the reality.[1] Where a unity that is constituted by the dynamics of social interactions—body language, eye contact, social signs—may be baffling to someone who struggles to participate in such social signification, the image of the church as a temple made up of many stones or a body made up of many organs may be readily accessible. It is can be represented using LEGO, which has proven value as an educational medium for adaptation and development in persons with autism:[2] one can imagine building a temple from individual blocks and communicating the significance of each person who is part of the church. Similarly, it can be represented by pointing to a plant or an animal that has differently shaped parts within its unified form: point to a dog or to a tree and one has found a solid visual parallel to what Paul says about the body of Christ with many members, and Jesus says about the vine with many branches. Each congregation of the church should reflect on whether it

seeks to nurture Christian unity by paying sustained attention
to these biblical images, or by social practices and customs that
are well-intentioned but are counterproductive or isolating for
autistic people. In these cases, far from helping autistic persons
to belong, the church may make them feel ever more out of place
within the community of faith. Furthermore, as the next two
observations will begin to highlight, the kind of unity that they
foster may be vulnerable to the particular value judgments (on
who belongs and who does not, or on who is important and who
is less so) that Paul disavows as "according to the flesh."

Second, the unity or solidarity that is identified in each of
these images is a function of the collective union between individual believers and Jesus Christ. Rather than solidarity principally being generated by the dynamic of personal interactions,
shared practices, and common beliefs, it is generated by the
union that binds each believer to Jesus in such a way that they
are described as being "in Christ." The practices that reflect or
depict this solidarity *derive* their significance from the unity that
they enact, rather than themselves generating the unity (even if,
in practice, they may consolidate or nurture it).

The point is illustrated by another of the very solid images
that is used by Paul to depict shared Christian identity, that of
putting on an item of clothing:

> ²⁷ As many of you as were baptized into Christ have clothed
> yourselves with Christ. ²⁸ There is no longer Jew or Greek,
> there is no longer slave or free, there is no longer male and
> female; for all of you are one in Christ Jesus. (Gal 3:27-28)

Everyone who wears clothes can comprehend or visualize without difficulty the image of clothing one reality (ourselves) with
another (Christ). It is potentially a vivid way of explaining to
a child or convert how their lives look different on the basis of
their new relationship with Christ, while also requiring them to
consider what it means to clothe themselves with a person and

his identity, and not just a sweater. For those with autism, whose sensory issues might have caused them to experience clothing as something that feels strange, it is an image that might be suggestive on multiple levels, or in relation to multiple senses. For Paul, a key element of the image's significance is that what each individual within the community has put on is the same thing: each has put on Christ. The fact that believers undergo a common ritual of identification, baptism, is also associated with this. Every person who is baptized wears the same single item of clothing: Christ. This transcends all particularities of ethnicity or gender (Jew and Greek, male and female), but also those of experience or status (slave or free). Such particularities are not erased: Paul's letters continue to be marked by references to the personal particularities of his addressees, who still bear male or female names and still carry their historical ethnic identities with them in those names. But the reality of union with Christ, which is made real by the presence of the Holy Spirit, is more basic to the corporate identity of believers than any of these particularities.

The point is an important one: "belonging" to the church is not a function of one's capacity to perform a certain kind of identity, with a complex of associated beliefs, and neither is it something that needs to be *felt* or perceived in order to be real. It is something that is constituted outside of our own consciousness by our union with Christ. It is objectively real, even when not perceived subjectively. Some discussion within the discipline of practical theology has highlighted the distinction between the concept of "belonging" and "inclusion" or "inclusivity": the latter words are popularly used in a positive way to indicate the intentional commitment of communities to show acceptance toward people who differ from the communal norms in some way. The concept of inclusion tends to be centered on authority, however, and to reflect an institutional way of thinking, rather than simply participation in a community. Leaders decide to impose "inclusive" policies, and what we are included within is generally the institution that they lead; "belonging" to a community, by contrast, is a matter of one's identification with the group, regardless, in a sense, of whether the leadership or structures of the group acknowledge one's existence or membership.[3] For the same reason, one may "belong" to a group even when marked by behaviors or characteristics that the institution or leadership of the group does not like: while the leadership may set the limits of the group's inclusivity, true "belonging" transcends such judgments. A person with autism may belong to the body of Christ without their status being officially endorsed. This is important for those who have faced, or whose children have faced, exclusion or marginalization by their fellow Christians. Having been asked to leave a church does not mean that you have ceased to be part of the body of Christ. Those who have asked you to leave, in fact, are the ones whose actions contradict the basic realities of the gospel.

Third, the images in question move beyond a general significance in relation to belonging to a much more specific significance in relation to the ascription of worth and how this is determined by our union with Christ, understood to involve the union of each person with the one God. Paul's elaboration of the body image in 1 Corinthians 12, for example, moves from a general sense of what it means to belong to a diversely composed but singular body into a more detailed account of how people who are different ought to value each other:

> [12] For just as the body is one and has many members, and all the members of the body, though many, are one body, so it is with Christ. [13] For in the one Spirit we were all baptized into one body—Jews or Greeks, slaves or free—and we were all made to drink of one Spirit.
> [14] Indeed, the body does not consist of one member but of many. [15] If the foot would say, "Because I am not a hand, I do

not belong to the body," that would not make it any less a part of the body. [16] And if the ear would say, "Because I am not an eye, I do not belong to the body," that would not make it any less a part of the body. [17] If the whole body were an eye, where would the hearing be? If the whole body were hearing, where would the sense of smell be? [18] But as it is, God arranged the members in the body, each one of them, as he chose. [19] If all were a single member, where would the body be? [20] As it is, there are many members, yet one body. [21] The eye cannot say to the hand, "I have no need of you," nor again the head to the feet, "I have no need of you." [22] On the contrary, the members of the body that seem to be weaker are indispensable, [23] and those members of the body that we think less honorable we clothe with greater honor, and our less respectable members are treated with greater respect; [24] whereas our more respectable members do not need this. But God has so arranged the body, giving the greater honor to the inferior member, [25] that there may be no dissension within the body, but the members may have the same care for one another. [26] If one member suffers, all suffer together with it; if one member is honored, all rejoice together with it. (1 Cor 12:12-26)

The passage opens with a reiteration of the point that we saw made above in Galatians: all who are baptized into Christ are clothed with a single shared reality that is more basic than the particularities of their identities. Interestingly, here this is linked to the singularity of the Holy Spirit who has been drunk by the members of the body.[4] In fact, the expression "one Spirit" reflects a pattern that has developed through 1 Corinthians from 8:6 onwards of rendering the unity of the church in a way that is conditioned by the classic statement of God's own oneness, the Shema of Deuteronomy 6:4.

> Hear, O Israel: The Lord our God, the Lord is one.
> (Deut 6:4, NIV)

In 1 Corinthians, this is first expanded to indicate that Jesus is included within the unique and singular identity of God:

Yet for us there is one God, the Father, from whom are all things and for whom we exist, and one Lord, Jesus Christ, through whom are all things and through whom we exist. (1 Cor 8:6)

This sets a pattern for what follows in subsequent chapters as the clothing of the members of the church with the identity of Jesus causes them to be included in this oneness:

> [16] The cup of blessing that we bless, is it not a sharing in the blood of Christ? The bread that we break, is it not a sharing in the body of Christ? [17] Because there is one bread, we who are many are one body, for we all partake of the one bread. (1 Cor 10:16-17)

The language of "sharing" is important here. It is participatory language that is connected in Greek to the idea of "fellowship":[5] because we are *partnered* to Jesus in the gospel, his reality determines and constitutes ours. We share in what he is, including his own participation in the oneness of God, a unity that now extends into the life of the church. When, in 1 Corinthians 12:13, this partnership is linked to the one Spirit's role in our baptism and to our collective drinking of this one Spirit, it is a further extension of the pattern of reflection on the oneness of God, linked to the consequent oneness of the church.

Conceptually, this is important to all that will follow. When members of the body of Christ are summoned to recognize their mutual interdependence and shared status in relation to God, it is on the basis of their participation in the life of the one God. It is, effectively, an expression of the Shema. Their unity is not a function of agreement or of common practice, although these are obviously (if not *inevitably*) corollaries of it, but of the formal bond that exists between the one God and his people through Christ.

This particularly positive implication of collective union with Christ brings with it a particularly negative implication for the way we typically pass value judgments on the status of fellow believers or other members of the church. We noted in chapter 3 that the gospel challenges worldly value systems and does so through the inversion of normal human expectations, particularly in relation to the cross and to election. As we saw there, the concept of "gift" is particularly important to the representation of salvation, but not in quite the way that we assume as moderns. It is not *just* the case that God gives the gift of salvation to those who do not deserve it—he does, but the notion of a "gift" in the ancient world did not automatically carry the connotation that the recipient did not merit such an action—but rather that the gift is given to those who lack, within themselves, all capacity to return what has been invested in them.[6] It is significant that 1 Corinthians 12, as it builds toward its statement that "we were all made to drink of one Spirit" (12:13),[7] throws around the vocabulary of gift and giving lavishly: the gift of salvation is given in a way that generates the community of the body of Christ, but even here our native tendency to ascribe capital value to certain kinds of activity or *charisma* and not to others can lead us to evaluate in a sinful way. Paul's intent throughout 1 Corinthians 12 is precisely to challenge such a tendency by pointing to the essential unity of the body as the purpose for which such gifts were given, and by locating this within the "gracedness" of all Christian existence.

We need to recognize our native tendency to admire or even idolize those who are impressively "gifted": great preachers and teachers, great worship leaders, or even just those Christians who have the ability to be funny and socially engaging. We also need to recognize that this natural response to such social qualities is so profound within our flesh that it will affect the ways that we think about unity itself: we will tend to see unity as something that is realized when we interact in socially accepted bonding practices—handshakes, eye contact, hugs, and so on—or in the performance of social identity through shared jargon or group-specific practices, such as the particular practices of prayer that characterize the tradition to which we belong. We will tend to think of unity as something that happens as a result of—or is realized in—the social things that we do; any who do not participate in these the way we expect them to are considered peripheral to the unity of the church, or even as a threat to that unity. In some cases, these members of the body of Christ may be marginalized or even excluded—the equivalent of the eye saying to the hand, "I have no need of you" (1 Cor 12:21)—because they do not perform the expected pattern of Christian social identity. They may even feel marginal because they do not fit that pattern—the equivalent of the foot saying, "Because I am not a hand, I do not belong to the body" (1 Cor 12:15).

It is important to recognize that Paul's logic does not represent the oneness of the body as the goal of Christian practice, but as its basis. The foot may consider itself not to belong to the body because it is different from the hand, *but it is wrong to do so.* The eye may think it has no need of the hand, *but it is wrong to do so.* The membership of foot and hand is not dependent upon the perceptions and practices of the members themselves, but upon the integrity of the organism in its union with Christ. Those who feel marginal or peripheral are confronted by this truth: they are more vitally part of the body of Christ than they (or anyone else) realize. Those who marginalize others are confronted by this truth: they are treating with disdain (even if unwittingly) a unity that derives from the oneness of God himself. This will underpin the principles that follow in this chapter.

Communication and Truthfulness in the Body of Christ

What we have just considered summons us to reflect on whether our social practices within the church are genuinely aligned with the reality that we are collectively united to Christ. It is a striking feature of the New Testament—though one that must be identified as an extension of the principles found in the Hebrew Bible—that the community is characterized by the practice of love. The rich description of the body of Christ in 1 Corinthians 12 is followed by Paul's famous description of love in 1 Corinthians 13. In order to highlight the connection between the two chapters, I include in the quotation that follows the last line of chapter 12:

> 12:31 But strive for the greater gifts. And I will show you a still more excellent way.
> 13:1 If I speak in the tongues of mortals and of angels, but do not have love, I am a noisy gong or a clanging cymbal. 2 And if I have prophetic powers, and understand all mysteries and all knowledge, and if I have all faith, so as to remove mountains, but do not have love, I am nothing. 3 If I give away all my possessions, and if I hand over my body so that I may boast, but do not have love, I gain nothing.
> 4 Love is patient; love is kind; love is not envious or boastful or arrogant 5 or rude. It does not insist on its own way; it is not irritable or resentful; 6 it does not rejoice in wrongdoing, but rejoices in the truth. 7 It bears all things, believes all things, hopes all things, endures all things. (1 Cor 12:31–13:7)

There is more to this description, of course, and much of it might be considered relevant to our thinking about autism, since it speaks about the limits of our present state of knowledge and of our openness to a radically different future. The point highlighted here, though, is that love is represented as crucial to the proper life of the body, as the members care for each other in ways that are patient, kind, humble, and generous.

A similar association is made by Jesus in John's Gospel, as the image of the vine and its branches leads to the command to practice love:

> 5 I am the vine, you are the branches. Those who abide in me and I in them bear much fruit, because apart from me you can do nothing. . . . 9 As the Father has loved me, so I have loved

you; abide in my love. [10] If you keep my commandments, you will abide in my love, just as I have kept my Father's commandments and abide in his love. [11] I have said these things to you so that my joy may be in you, and that your joy may be complete.

[12] "This is my commandment, that you love one another as I have loved you." (John 15:5, 9-12)

Again, more could be quoted and more could be said about it, but the simple point is that the imagery that speaks of the unity of the body, always as a function of its collective union with Christ, is linked to the commandment to love one another. That commandment, of course, can be seen as a development of the command to love one's neighbor, which is a corollary of the command to love the one God (Mark 12:29-31 and parallels, drawing on Deut 6:4 and Lev 19:18).

What is easily overlooked is that this command entails a commitment to practicing "truthfulness." This emerges very clearly in 1 Corinthians 13:6, where love "rejoices in the truth." The connection is also visible in a number of other texts, several of which are from the Johannine corpus:

Now that you have purified your souls by your obedience to the truth so that you have genuine mutual love, love one another deeply from the heart. (1 Pet 1:22)

Little children, let us love, not in word or speech, but in truth and action. (1 John 3:18)

The elder to the elect lady and her children, whom I love in the truth, and not only I but also all who know the truth. (2 John 1:1)

Grace, mercy, and peace will be with us from God the Father and from Jesus Christ, the Father's Son, in truth and love. (2 John 3)

The elder to the beloved Gaius, whom I love in truth. (3 John 1:1)

Perhaps the most striking of all texts, given what we have seen, is Ephesians 4:15:

> But speaking the truth in love, we must grow up in every way into him who is the head, into Christ.

Love, then, is inseparable from truth, and "truthfulness" must be a property of those who love one another in the body of Christ. We are, of course, united to the one who *is* the truth (John 14:6) by the Spirit of Truth (John 14:17, 15:26).

The truthfulness of the believer is also a major theme in the Old Testament, especially in the Psalms (e.g., Pss 15:2, 51:6, 86:11; cf. Ps 5:9) and in Proverbs (e.g., Prov 12:17, 23:23). Here it is consistently represented as a quality shared with God himself, the one who rides out victoriously in the cause of truth and meekness (Ps 45:4).

Recognizing this is important, because much of our social practice is actually quite untruthful. We communicate in coded messages, sometimes by double entendre, or wear masks that hide our real thoughts or feelings; we perform social identities, often without being honest with ourselves that we are doing so. We have untruthful conventions, because we want to be perceived in socially favorable ways that will build our symbolic capital. Persons with autism are widely recognized to struggle with such conventions, although some are skilled at camouflaging their difficulties.[8] These conventions contribute to their own experience of marginalization, all while their own truthfulness—that socially inappropriate honesty that is commonly a feature of autism—is considered offensive, or is made the object of jokes or mockery. Recovering a serious commitment to the practice of truthfulness within the community of love is a necessary step in fostering the belonging of those with autism.

This is not to give those with autism free reign to be as offen-sively or as aggressively honest as they want: truthfulness must be conditioned by love, which means developing an awareness that certain expressions can cause hurt and learning how to communicate in ways that are edifying rather than destructive. But it does mean that the body of Christ collectively recognizes that it often embodies the deceptiveness of sin and that its per-ceptions of those with autism are often compromised by this. It means that we need to be repentant of our tendency to identify Christian love and unity with the performance of certain social expectations and need to reevaluate our responses to the sim-plicity of communication that is often associated with autism. It means, in short, allowing the presence of autism within the church to drive us to ask again, "What should living truthfully and lovingly in the body of Christ actually look like?"

Accommodating the Sensory Needs of Persons with Autism

The church is a sensory space, to an extent that persons with typical senses seldom register. Occasionally, perhaps, something may have an intense impact on those persons: feedback from the sound system or the smell of halitosis when talking to some-one may go through them with a sensory jolt. For most people, though, such things happen only occasionally and the sensory world quickly returns to normal. They do not register the smell of a hair product, the gain settings on the amplifier, the kind of lighting that has been fitted, or the layout of the seating as mat-ters that will bear on the well-being of others in the church. For a person with autism, however, each of these elements—and a myriad more beside—has the potential to cause extreme sensory distress. The perfume that one person loves wearing, perhaps because of its emotional associations for them, is painful to the person with autism, who may not even be sitting near them in the church. Wearing that perfume may be an act of gratitude to the person who gave it, but it is unwittingly an act of violence to another member of the body of Christ, or to their child.

I put the issue in this way to highlight that a loving accommodation of the needs of others is necessary, and that this accommodation involves a willingness to forgo certain good and enjoyable things within certain sensory spaces. It involves, in other words, a willingness to constrain our freedoms out of concern for the good of others who may be hurt in some way by those freedoms.

The biblical passages that most clearly speak to this are those in which Paul speaks about the needs of "weaker" and "stronger" believers, notably Romans 14 and 15. Some care needs to be taken in applying these passages, since the weakness that is described there appears to be a characteristic of the believers' faith, and the specific issues involved are distinctively about abstention from certain practices. That is, Romans 14 and 15 are immediately about something quite different from the sensory situation that we are considering in relation to autism. Nonetheless, what they say is highly relevant to the sensory challenges associated with autism, provided we are careful in our reapplication from one issue to another.

The key to their relevance lies in the fact that they involve very specific applications of the principles of unity and value that we have outlined so far in this and the previous chapter. Note, for example, how the priority of God's election (here represented in the associated motif of his "welcome")[9] is brought to bear on the value judgments of those who despise others who act differently than themselves. Note also the emphasis on a common relationship that binds those who have different values, by which those who live and die are equally "the Lord's." The key expressions are highlighted below.

¹ Welcome (*proslambanesthe*) those who are weak in faith, but not for the purpose of quarreling over opinions. ² Some believe in eating anything, while the weak eat only vegetables. ³ Those who eat must not despise those who abstain, and those who abstain must not pass judgment on those who eat; *for God has welcomed* (*proselabeto*) *them.* ⁴ Who are you to pass judgment on servants of another? It is before their own lord that they stand or fall. And they will be upheld, for the Lord is able to make them stand.

⁵ Some judge one day to be better than another, while others judge all days to be alike. Let all be fully convinced in their own minds. ⁶ Those who observe the day, observe it in honor of the Lord. Also those who eat, eat in honor of the Lord, since they give thanks to God; while those who abstain, abstain in honor of the Lord and give thanks to God.

⁷ We do not live to ourselves, and we do not die to ourselves. ⁸ If we live, we live to the Lord, and if we die, we die to the Lord; so then, whether we live or whether we die, we are the Lord's. ⁹ For to this end Christ died and lived again, so that he might be Lord of both the dead and the living. (Rom 14:1-9)

Once the links between this and the theology of love that we have been considering are recognized, we can note a further important point that ties back to chapter 3. Paul frequently uses the binary of the weak and the strong in relation to the gospel's inversion of normal values, as he affirms the place of the "weak" within the community: God "chose the weak things of the world to shame the strong things" (1 Cor 1:27, my translation). This is part of a broader tendency to speak in positive terms about weakness as something through which the potent fullness of God makes itself visible: "we have this treasure in jars of clay, to show that the excess of power is of God, and not of ourselves" (2 Cor 4:7, my translation). The point of note is that we will tend to assume that Romans 14 and 15 represent the "weaker brother" as deficient or, in some sense, lesser than the stronger counterpart; ironically, perhaps, we can pass a judgment of sorts when we do so. But when the language of strength and weakness is read against its wider background in Paul, it takes on a set of connotations that actually tie more closely to the logic of Romans 14 and 15. Those who are weak are no less (or, perhaps better, no *lesser*) a part of the body than those who are strong; they must be treated with equal respect and not despised, and their needs must be accommodated with love. Again, I have highlighted some particularly relevant language in Romans 14:

> [13] Let us therefore no longer pass judgment on one another, but resolve instead never to put a stumbling block or hindrance in the way of another. [14] I know and am persuaded in the Lord Jesus that nothing is unclean in itself; but it is unclean for anyone who thinks it unclean. [15] *If your brother or sister is being injured by what you eat, you are no longer walking in love.* Do not let what you eat cause the ruin of one for whom Christ died. [16] So do not let your good be spoken of as evil. [17] For the kingdom of God is not food and drink but righteousness and peace and joy in the Holy Spirit. (Rom 14:13-17)

Such language extends into Romans 15, where it is rendered in terms of an obligation to set aside one's own preferences and prerogatives for the good of the "neighbor" and with a view to the harmony and unity of the Christian community.

> [1] We who are strong ought to put up with the failings of the weak, and not to please ourselves. [2] Each of us must please our neighbor for the good purpose of building up the neighbor. [3] For Christ did not please himself; but, as it is written, "The insults of those who insult you have fallen on me." [4] For whatever was written in former days was written for our instruction, so that by steadfastness and by the encouragement of the scriptures we might have hope. [5] May the God of steadfastness and encouragement grant you to live in harmony with one another, in accordance with Christ Jesus, [6] so that together you may with one voice glorify the God and Father of our Lord Jesus Christ. (Rom 15:1-6)

As I have stressed throughout this section, we are dealing with a part of Paul's writings that is directed toward the question of how Christians whose strength of conscience allows them to engage in certain activities ought to view other Christians whose weakness prohibits them from such engagement. Paul is not, in any obvious sense, talking about how Christians should react to the distinctive needs of those with autism. But there is a significant point of correspondence, because what underlies the obligation to behave in a particular way is the unity of the body of Christ and the status of its weak members as equally chosen and equally important within it. Whether the weakness is one of poverty, intellect, or faith, the principle is the same: this person belongs because of God's welcoming, and their needs must now be met with love by the community. "If one member suffers, all suffer together with it" (1 Cor 12:26).

For Paul, this means that the freedom of the gospel is constrained by the obligation to love. Elsewhere he will say, "'All things are lawful,' but not all things are beneficial. 'All things are lawful,' but not all things build up" (1 Cor 10:23; cf. 6:12). As the speech marks in the translation suggest, Paul is probably here quoting something widely said in defense of the Christian's freedom, but his response indicates that his readers have failed to recognize that this freedom is inseparable from the responsibility to build up the body of Christ in love. Christian freedom may be expressed in a willingness to forgo something, out of love for Christ and his members.

This "freedom to forgo" and obligation to accommodate the needs of others has significant bearing on how Christians participate in the life of the church. If there is a person with autism in the church, or if someone brings a person with autism *into* the church, they may come with sensory vulnerabilities that are unintentionally hurt by the actions of others, through the decision to use certain cosmetic products or turn the PA system up. Given the variation that characterizes autism, some of these problems cannot be anticipated and can only be dealt with reactively: it is only once we have learned that something is triggering a problem that we can do anything about it. Parents, for example, may eventually have to share with someone what their autistic child has told them about the effects of their favorite deodorant. An adult may eventually have to explain to a friend why he screws up his face in his presence. Having said this, it is important that all churches make their members aware of the sensory challenges associated with autism, for two reasons. First, the inevitable conversations about sensory reactions will be less likely to cause offense if there is an awareness within the culture that such reactions are common, if atypical. If Christians generally know that autism involves hard-to-predict sensory issues, they are less likely to be offended or upset when they are told by a parent, caregiver, friend, or pastor that their actions are contributing to these. Second, the more awareness there is about sensory issues in autism, the more likely it is that people will make choices that accommodate the recognition that certain things are common triggers. If more Christians knew about sensory issues, perhaps fewer of them would wear perfumes or strong deodorants to church, for example; or perhaps the church would recognize the need to purchase unfragranced hand soaps.[10]

There are two further issues that need to be mentioned, as a kind of flip side to what we have been discussing. First, those with profound autism may themselves contribute in challenging ways to the sensory environment of the church. They may scream, shout, and generally behave in quite disruptive ways. This, too, must be accommodated in love. Since beginning my work on autism, I have read numerous testimonies of Christian families who have been asked to leave churches because of the behavior of their autistic child, and various reports have highlighted how widespread a problem this is.[11] The problem is often that this behavior disrupts a particular culture of what church worship should look like; interestingly, this may be less of a problem in certain traditional forms of worship (such as Eastern Orthodox services) than it is in evangelical churches, which tend to expect that services will be slicker. The exclusion of Christians because of their difficult contributions to the sensory environment of the church is a serious problem, for all of the reasons noted above: "If one member suffers, all suffer together with it."

It may be worth bearing in mind that worship in the early church probably looked quite different than what we are familiar with today. For one thing, many members of the early church were from the poverty classes or were even slaves; such people had little control over their own lives and the timing of their activities. They were probably unable to schedule a Sunday in such a way that they could arrive in time for the prechurch Bible study and then sit through the main service, leaving time afterwards to join others for coffee before heading home. Services were probably subject to a constant flux of attendance, with interruptions of sorts throughout. The descriptions we do have of worship in the New Testament do not provide us with anything definitive by way of a description, but they do not sound particularly formulaic, even if they suggest *disorder* to be a bad thing (see, for example, 1 Cor 14:26-33). We tend to establish a certain pattern of worship and then identify this as the order that God wants to characterize his church, but there is a danger that we have created idols out of our traditions. How we react to the shout of an autistic child may well be a telling sign that we are hard-hearted idolaters and not softhearted worshipers.

Second, the principles that underlie the Christian obligation to accommodate the sensory needs of those with autism also bear on the autistic themselves. If my senses are hurt by the actions of others, I am obligated to treat them with love; I cannot despise them for their choice of cosmetics or their singing. This is more of an issue than might be recognized by those who are not autistic. Sensory overload can create a fragmented emotional and psychological state, leading to anger and other emotions; it can lead to a meltdown. Part of the formational development of the Christian with autism involves learning how to manage such emotions, and this involves resisting the tendency to direct that anger toward those who have been involved in the pain, often through no fault of their own. Of course, it also involves resisting the desire to abstain from all Christian fellowship.

The Busy Church and the Need for Decompression

A final point must now be made. Sensory and social experiences are often exhausting for autistic people and, consequently, also for those who care for them. They may enjoy them and value the fact that they participated in them, but they may need to recover from the experience in ways that others do not. The language that is often used by those with autism is that after such experiences they need to "decompress." The physical or physiological elements of a stress reaction have built up in their system, accompanied by the fatigue that results from the effort of processing the data, and their bodies and brains need to recover. Sometimes a measure of decompression can be achieved through "stimming" behaviors of one kind or another, even when in the midst of the social or sensory experience.[12] Often, though, the person needs to be left alone for a lengthy period of time.

This can be difficult to understand for those who are naturally gregarious or who might be defined as extroverts. It can also be difficult to understand for those whose role within a church makes them particularly invested in seeing high numbers present at each activity and identifying those numbers with success. Often the two groups are identical, where those who perform the role of church leader are naturally social and identify the unity of the church with social activities. The issue is compounded by what we have talked about already in this book: we tend to be very focused on the performance of identity that our culture considers to be the marker of a group insider, and frequency of attendance at services is often an element of this. The person who attends fewer services may not be considered an outsider, but may be seen as marginal or uncommitted, less important or less valuable than the person who attends many, who will be seen as a key member of the church.

Church leaders often have no awareness of the kind of pressure they put on members of their congregations to attend multiple activities each week, or even throughout the course of a Sunday. They are often themselves unaware of the extent to which they pass judgment on the value of attendees. It is particularly important that they understand the need of those with autism to recover from social and sensory activities, and the danger of not respecting that need. Real damage can be done to those who are not given appropriate time to recover from the experience of attending church. It is equivalent to an athlete overtraining: the physiological damage can be counterproductive and can often take a long time to heal.

This may, in turn, invite some reflection on whether church schedules are simply too busy, perhaps because they have developed largely to serve the preferences of the gregarious neurotypical. This is perhaps a point where the principle of Sabbath needs to be reclaimed more seriously for the Christian tradition. The principle of Sabbath is rest; for Jews, the Sabbath is "a period of sacred stasis" when they participate in (and do not simply imitate) the rest of God himself.[13] Our Sundays are often hectic, busy times, and some thrive on the social energy that they involve; for those with autism, the possibility of recovering a sacred time in which we genuinely rest from the social and sensory demands of the world may be deeply attractive.

Conclusions

Churches are social and sensory spaces. For those whose social and sensory profiles or capacities are "normal," the significance of this will not be perceived; it will be processed at a tacit level. Those who struggle to participate in such spaces, however, will be painfully aware of the factors at work, and their difficulties will often make them objects of exclusion for the "normal." They will be marginalized, either incidentally or deliberately, by their limited ability to participate in the environment of the church. If the "furniture" of that environment were prescribed by God, then perhaps this would be *their* problem, rather than anyone else's. But, as we have seen, *their* problem is the church's problem—if one part of the body suffers, all do—and what they struggle with is often the performance of a worldly culture, rather than the practicing of genuinely biblical worship.

The images of the church as a corporate unity—the body, the temple, the vine—provide concrete pictures that should be the object of sustained reflection by the church as it seeks to understand its nature in Christ. For those with autism, such concrete images can provide a much stronger basis for perceiving their "belonging" to the church than the social practices of the neurotypical. For churches, these can be the basis for a sense of repentance over practices that have been well intentioned but have excluded or marginalized many.

Crucially, many of the church's practices are absolutely fine in themselves, but prove to be problematic for persons with autism. This is true of collective activities and of personal ones.

Paul's teaching on the weak and the strong, while itself principally concerned with the limiting of moral freedoms out of love, provides us with a means to consider the responsibility to forgo certain things out of concern for the needs of the weak. Such things may be social or they may be sensory; the decision to forgo them is an act of love, shown to those who would be injured in some sense by our practicing of freedoms, even if the freedom is simply to wear cosmetic products.

5

THE DARK SIDE OF AUTISM

Anxiety, Depression, and Addiction

Autism brings challenges, and it is important that we do not lose sight of these while challenging attitudes toward autistic persons within the church. As part of this, we need to recognize the common association of autism with related conditions such as anxiety, depression, and addiction. These conditions are hardly unique to persons with autism, but they present in distinctive ways for those with the condition and generate particular personal and pastoral challenges. I am conscious that some readers will themselves be autistic and may bring some painful experience to their reading of this chapter; I hope that what is written here will be comforting on certain levels and constructively helpful on others. I am conscious, too, of the fact that pastors may read this in an effort to understand the distinctive challenges that accompany autism. For them, I want to emphasize the need to understand the factors that may make these associated problems particularly difficult for autistic people, and that may require pastors to implement different strategies to address the problems than they would use with others. I also want to emphasize, though, the need to engage with autistic persons *as persons*, and to recognize that each will embody autism differently. There is a real pastoral danger of assuming that every person with autism struggles with addiction or with depression and then engaging with them in ways that reflect this assumption. This chapter is not intended to support such assumptions, but to highlight the relative co-occurrence (or comorbidity)[1] of such conditions with autism and to consider some of the biblical material that might be brought to bear upon it. I will begin by outlining some of the research onto addiction and other problems; I will consider them separately, though of course they may cluster together and overlap.

Autism, Anxiety, and Depression

It is well established in the scientific literature that autism often co-occurs with anxiety and/or depression, both of which are really umbrella terms for a range of conditions and experiences (as distinct from being things in their own right, with a particular form). Some estimates have placed the level of co-occurrence as high as 85 percent, although more recent research has suggested those figures may have been overestimated.[2] The co-occurrence of diagnosed conditions is certainly statistically significant, however: some reviews have found that 29 percent of those diagnosed with autism are also diagnosed with anxiety, and 25 percent of those diagnosed with autism also have a diagnosis of depression.[3] Of course, these are figures associated with actual diagnosis; the prevalence of anxiety and depression among those with autism is likely to be significantly higher than is indicated by these figures, since the symptoms may not present to a level that would be diagnosed clinically as anxiety or depression. One recent study reports that 46 percent of persons with autism experience moderate to severe anxiety and 44 percent experience depression. It is worth noting that one of the key studies often cited in relation to this establishes a link between autism and the elevated presence of a wide range of other health issues, such as gastrointestinal disorders and sleep disorders,[4] but depression and anxiety are the most prevalent associated conditions, by a huge margin.

It is important to recognize just how serious the effects of anxiety and depression can be for those with autism. Croen et al. noticed a statistically significant elevation of attempted suicide rates among those with autism:

> Of particular concern is the fivefold higher rate of diagnosed suicide attempts we observed among adults with ASD compared to controls. Nearly half of the adults with ASD with a diagnosis of attempted suicide did not also have a diagnosis of depression, suggesting that depression may be underdiagnosed in the autistic population, resulting in lack of needed treatment.[5]

This finding is broadly supported by a number of other studies. We must be careful, of course, not to assume that every person with autism will have suicidal thoughts, either now or in the future, but we must also be aware that the mental health problems that often occur with autism can be of a particularly severe kind.

It is also important to recognize how little is currently known about the factors that underlie these comorbidities. While it is probably the case that the distinctive neurological development of the person with autism is among these, there may also be external factors that play a role in the actual occurrence of the condition. Some of these factors may be dramatic (such as bullying or trauma), but others may be quite mundane, such as circumstances that require the person with autism to behave differently from their preferred routine and that disrupt the sameness of their environment.[6] The cumulative effects of sensory overload and social exhaustion are also, of course, important factors. Researchers acknowledge that more work needs to be done on the specific ways in which these factors bear on comorbidity and recognize that this bears on the use of medication to treat both anxiety and depression in persons with autism:

> Psychopharmacological treatment has received the most attention with respect to mood disorders. Treatment focuses on symptom reduction, but there is limited evidence for efficacy in the ASD population.[7]

The treatment of depression and anxiety—and other psychopathologies that occur together with autism—will never be as simple as administering a medicine (although medication *may* prove valuable). It will always involve a complex of social and environmental adaptations, including within the environment of the church.

Alongside this, the pressure of caring for those with autism may itself create pastoral needs. Depression and anxiety have also been widely observed in those involved in the long-term care of autistic people, and those committed to acting in love for persons with autism need to be aware that those around them—their families and caregivers, or their spouses—may quietly carry their own burden of hidden pain, perhaps even compounded by a sense of guilt at the way they feel.

Autism and Addiction

The evidence for the co-occurrence of autism and addiction disorders has grown in recent years, from a fairly large body of somewhat anecdotal evidence (often circulating within the autism support communities)[8] to a more precise body of scientific research. Some of this research indicates a higher incidence of substance abuse among those with autism than among the wider population;[9] other research indicates similarly higher levels of non–substance-based addictions, such as internet addictions of various sorts.[10] These studies, which often involve large cohorts and have emerged from a range of different cultural contexts, provide statistical support for what has long been known within the support communities associated with autism: addictions often accompany the condition and constitute a distinct challenge that needs to be cared for properly.

We need to be careful as we seek to understand why addiction often co-occurs with autism, because the causative factors may be complex. This will have a significant bearing on how the addictions in question might be understood and, perhaps, treated.

One significant factor is the anxiety that also co-occurs in autism. As we have seen, some studies suggest that a high percentage of those with autism also experience significant levels of anxiety, in which the sensory environment and the difficulty of establishing control over the world around us play a significant role. Some of the substance use associated with autism is considered to be a form of "self-medication"; alcohol, in particular, is used as a means to relax, to slow or soften the processing of sensory input, or bring a stressed body into something approaching a restful state. We know, of course, that excessive use of alcohol does not sustain relaxation and creates further physiological problems, but, for a brief period, it will allow a person with autism to enjoy some respite from the overwhelming anxiety that they may feel much of the time. Something similar can be said about sensory or social overload: the person may not have been consciously anxious, but may have been overstimulated in other ways and is now physiologically stressed, with elevated cortisol levels and the other typical markers of stress. Alcohol or other substances provide a means to feel more relaxed, for a while at least. Aside from anxiety and overload, substances can also provide a means simply to slow down the sheer speed of thought that autistic people often experience.

This same causative factor might play a part in non-substance addictions, particularly those connected with the internet. This can provide a means of escape from the sensory and social world that creates anxiety or overload; it is accessed on the terms of the user, allowing a sense of control, and its sensory elements are limited and manageable. As with substances, however, it can interact in dangerous ways with our highly plastic brains, particularly the parts that are often referred to as our "reward circuitry."[11] Simply put, our brains are designed to deal with a certain amount of data flow and to decide which of those data (especially new ones) are rewarding and worth continuing to pursue; the rate of data flow associated with the internet is powerfully hyperstimulating, something increasingly recognized to be a factor in addiction to high-speed pornography,[12] but also a factor in internet addiction more broadly. Persons turn to the internet feeling like they are in control of their clicks, but very quickly that relationship flips.

There are also explanatory accounts for the co-occurrence of addiction and autism that recognize the extent to which the autistic brain, or even the autistic physiology, may be more vulnerable to substance addiction than that of the nonautistic person. Those with autism typically prefer routine and repetition—habit—and a regular practice of using a particular substance or performing a particular activity may quickly become part of their mental furniture. If the use is modest, this may not be a problem, but if it becomes more extreme, then it can be very damaging. Some research has also suggested that there are overlapping molecular and physiological factors in autism spectrum disorders and addictions. The same protein distributions have been observed in the development of autism that are seen in addictive drug responses, and the same atypical characteristics of the reward pathways in the brain are also observable in both.[13]

For some with autism, a very different factor may be involved. Although it tends to be overshadowed in perceptions of autism by *hyper*sensitivity, some with autism are *hypo*sensitive; they do not experience stimulation until the stimulant is excessively present. They need to be hyperstimulated in order to feel something. Certain substances, or certain practices, may trigger the reward circuitry because they bring about an enjoyable state of stimulation that is not experienced by normal means.

Taken together, these observations should foster a better pastoral response to the experience of addiction in relation to autism. Without suggesting that that addiction should go unchallenged or unaddressed, they help to explain why it can be such a significant feature of the experience of those with autism, and they inform a more realistic understanding of what behavioral change might involve. For those who are autistic and have dealt with addiction throughout their lives, the observations may bring a deep sense of relief, even as they throw the challenge of breaking patterns of addiction into a new light. We are not freed from our responsibility to take ownership of our actions, but we do have some sense of *why* it is so particularly difficult for us to break free of these behaviors. For their friends and family or for pastors, these observations may lead to a kinder response to often destructive behaviors.

The Gospel as the Context

We must begin by affirming that the gospel recontextualizes all such experiences. It is the determinative framework within which we must consider them. This is no insignificant claim: in it we affirm that there is a truth that conditions the significance of our weaknesses and prohibits us from thinking about them in isolation. When we think about anxiety, depression, suicide, and addiction in isolation, they are simply terrible and hopeless things. When we set them within the framework of the gospel, their awfulness may not be diminished, but it is no longer the last or definitive word that may be spoken about them. They are framed by mercy and hope.

Most importantly, we affirm that Jesus Christ and not our personal experience is the rock of our salvation. We are saved by grace through him. Our salvation does not rest upon the stability of our minds or upon our performance of obedience, or even upon the quality of our faith, but upon him and upon his work. As we participate in him, our minds may come to enjoy stability, and we may learn obedience, but these will never become the basis for our salvation; he and he alone is that basis.

This should be a genuinely and immensely comforting truth. The prospects for our future are not limited by the weakness of our selves, and the flesh in which they are embodied, but by his potency. This why Paul contrasts the emptiness or nastiness of the righteousness that is "of myself" with the perfection of the righteousness "of God" that is found in "knowing Christ" (Phil 3:9, my translation). The righteousness that he knows now has its origin not just in an action outside of himself (i.e., the self-sacrifice of Jesus on the cross), but in a person whose personal presence now constitutes that righteousness within him.

My salvation originates outside of myself, in the person of Jesus Christ; it is really present in me through the Spirit, even if my weak flesh is still compromised in its awareness of this truth. My body is not yet fully redeemed, and it groans along with the rest of the cosmos at the truth of that condition (Rom 8:22-27); it is only because the Spirit is in me that I can have any trust in my status as a child of God (Rom 8:16). I am still perishable and inglorious, but look forward to the day when I am entirely spiritual, in every atom of my body (1 Cor 15:44). My faith is simply the means by which I enjoy this reality; it is not the reality itself. My faith can be weak and fickle, but this does not detract from the reality that it allows me to enjoy.

When we recognize not just that we are forgiven through Christ, but that the entire grounds of our life and hope lie in him, outside the limits of our own selves, everything changes. I am an addict, and it is important that I face up to that reality, but something more basic defines who I am and forms the basis of my inclusion in God's kingdom. I am darkened by depression to the point where I see no hope of eternal life, but the certainty of that life is not compromised by the limits of my mental state. I am anxious, but my limited capacity to trust unfailingly that the situation is in God's hands does not cause him to drop the world with a shrug. Recognizing the priority and exteriority of God's grace in Christ is a vital pastoral starting point to dealing with the challenging realities of autism.[14]

There are various points in the New Testament that seem to project the reality of the gospel both back and forward through eternity. Christ is the firstborn of all creation, through whom and for whom all things were made and in whom they hold together (Col 1:16-17); he is the one in whom we were chosen before the foundation of the world (Eph 1:4), foreknown before the foundation of the world, but revealed in these end-times. Depending on how we translate the verse, he may even be described as the Lamb that was slain before the foundation of the world (Rev 13:8).[15] These verses all recognize that the temporally particular events of the life, death, resurrection, and ascension of Jesus are events associated with the temporally transcendent life of the eternal God. They bear materially on every moment of God's dealing with the cosmos and its inhabitants, including each moment of weakness embodied by us. This is a truth more basic, more comprehensive, than that of our sins and failures.

This bears on every aspect of autism, and underpins what follows, but I want to note here one very specific application of this truth. As we noted, rates of attempted suicide are considerably higher among persons with autism than among the wider

population; it may well be the case that some actual deaths from
suicide are connected to undiagnosed autism. Pastorally, this
can bring all kinds of dismal pain to everyone involved. I recall
the comments made by a friend of mine, a pastor called Angus
Macrae who is currently the moderator of the Free Church of
Scotland, after someone in his congregation committed suicide
and he had the painful experience of presiding over the funeral:
"You can lose a battle but win the war, even if, for some soldiers,
the battle is their last." The war is won, and always has been, but
the battles are real, and some do not survive them. Participation
in the victory is not confined to those who see its final realization
on earth, but to all whose death takes place in union with Christ,
even if their personal defeat took place in a moment of darkness
when their faith quailed.

> If we are faithless, he remains faithful —
>   for he cannot deny himself. (2 Tim 2:13)

For those processing the loss of someone to suicide, this may
bring little immediate comfort, but it may allow some healing
and hope to emerge in time.

We Have a Great High Priest

As part of our affirmation of the gospel as the context in which
to consider the challenges of autism, we also need to appreciate
the significance of Jesus' status as the "great high priest."

> [14] Since, then, we have a great high priest who has passed
> through the heavens, Jesus, the Son of God, let us hold fast
> to our confession. [15] For we do not have a high priest who is
> unable to sympathize with our weaknesses, but we have one
> who in every respect has been tested as we are, yet without sin.
> (Heb 4:14-15)

Hebrews represents Jesus as the high priest who ministers in
the heavenly sanctuary, the real temple after which the earthly

one is patterned.[16] The author represents Jesus as constituting the true reality that the various elements of the earthly cult figurally signify:[17] he is the high priest, but he is also the offering that the high priest brings as a sacrifice, and his sacrificial significance absorbs several of the offerings listed in the Torah.[18]

The author emphasizes two issues that are of particular relevance to the challenges constituted by autism. First, this high priest shares our human nature, with all its frailties and with all the temptations that accompany those frailties. He himself remains without sin, but his sharing of our nature means that he is able to minister in our behalf and to help us in our weakness:

> [17] For this reason he had to be made like his brothers in every way, in order that he might become a merciful and faithful high priest in service to God, and that he might make atonement for the sins of the people. [18] Because he himself was tested (or "tempted," *peirastheis*) by what he suffered, he is able to help those who are being tested (or "tempted," *peirazomenois*). (Heb 2:17-18, NIV, 1984 ed.)

> He is able to deal gently with the ignorant and wayward, since he himself is subject to weakness. (Heb 5:2)

It needs to be stressed repeatedly that Jesus involves himself in our lives as one who has lived the reality of human weakness and the suffering that accompanies it. Even if he himself never allowed temptation to become sin, he deals sympathetically with those who live out that same condition of weakness and vulnerability. He is gentle with them—with us—in a way that is so important for all who deal pastorally with those whose wounds, even if self-inflicted, are raw.

Second, through the perfection of the sacrifice that he has offered, this sympathetic high priest has removed every obstacle to fellowship with God. Here it is important to grasp that the sacrificial imagery used in Hebrews does not solely or even principally represent atonement in terms of penal substitution.

That idea may be present, depending on how we understand 2:9 and 2:17, but penal substitution focuses on the concept of punishment or penalty, where Hebrews is much more oriented toward the concept of the cleansing or purification that a sacrifice accomplishes. This, indeed, is emphasized in the opening lines of the book:

> When he had made purification for sins (*katharismon tōn hamartiōn poiēsamenos*), he sat down at the right hand of the Majesty on high. (Heb 1:3)

Through the course of the book, particularly in chapters 7–11, the author makes clear that Jesus' sacrifice has purified our consciences from our sins and has also purified the heavenly temple itself from all uncleanness:

> [13] For if the blood of goats and bulls, with the sprinkling of the ashes of a heifer, sanctifies those who have been defiled so that their flesh is purified, [14] how much more will the blood of Christ, who through the eternal Spirit offered himself without blemish to God, purify our conscience from dead works to worship the living God!

> [23] Thus it was necessary for the sketches of the heavenly things to be purified with these rites, but the heavenly things themselves need better sacrifices than these. [24] For Christ did not enter a sanctuary made by human hands, a mere copy of the true one, but he entered into heaven itself, now to appear in the presence of God on our behalf. (Heb 9:13-14, 23-24)

Such language of purity and impurity is, on one level, alien to much contemporary society. Unless we belong to religious communities that still maintain some concept of ritual impurity, the imagery can be difficult for us to grasp at a formal level. I stress it, however, because, at a deeper level, it resonates with the issues of self-image that accompany depression and addiction. Whether justified or not, and whether at a level we could articulate or not, we often perceive ourselves to be unclean. We may feel that we are, in some sense, tainted by our actions. Or, because our minds are in a state of dysfunction through anxiety or depression, we may *feel* unclean in ways that are difficult to trace logically and that are not, in fact, appropriate, yet are impossible to escape. This is not just an issue for those with autism but for many who experience mental health issues, including those whose problems are traced back to abuse or trauma. For all who have this deep sense of pollution, whether justified or not, the gospel account of Hebrews speaks powerfully of the right of access to the presence of God that has been secured for us by Jesus:

> [19] Therefore, my friends, since we have confidence to enter the sanctuary by the blood of Jesus, [20] by the new and living way that he opened for us through the curtain (that is, through his flesh), [21] and since we have a great priest over the house of God, [22] let us approach with a true heart in full assurance of faith, with our hearts sprinkled clean from an evil conscience and our bodies washed with pure water. [23] Let us hold fast to the confession of our hope without wavering, for he who has promised is faithful. [24] And let us consider how to provoke one another to love and good deeds, [25] not neglecting to meet together, as is the habit of some, but encouraging one another, and all the more as you see the Day approaching. (Heb 10:19-25)

Weakness and Metamorphosis

The Treasure of the Gospel and the Jars of Clay

The discussion at the beginning of this chapter highlighted that the challenges associated with autism emerge from the physical and neurophysiological realities of the person as they experience the social and sensory world.[19] These challenges assume a real moral significance: they participate in the higher-order moral realities that we speak of as "good" and "evil" and can appropriately be labeled with such language. But we must not lose sight of the physical and neurophysiological realities from which they emerge and upon which they bear. This is to recognize that they are distinctively associated with the particular *embodied* reality of the person with autism. They are associated with their "flesh."

We have seen already, in chapter 3, that the language of "the flesh" (*sarx*) is used by Paul to designate sin as a constitutional reality; it is not just something we do, but something that is in our nature, in our makeup. There we saw its relevance to the natural value system that comes from that nature, which *normally* ascribes worth and honor on the basis of perceived social capital and typically treats the autistic (along with all who differ from our norms) with disdain. This value system is held to account by the gospel of Jesus Christ and by his Spirit, but remains stubbornly persistent within his church. We also noted that those with autism are often freed from certain aspects of this, because their "neurotype" does not allow them to participate easily in the intuitive ascription of honor to the socially impressive.

There are, however, other ways in which the "fleshly" constitution of a person can cause them to act in ways that should be labeled quite properly as "sin," or to suffer things that should properly be called "evil." Each person has a different constitution, even if there is enough in common to speak of a shared human nature (the theological significance of this comment will emerge in due course). The physical constitution of a person with autism can give rise to a different set of problems than that of a "neurotypical" person. Both sets of problems, though, are associated with the "flesh," the physical and neurophysiological particularities of each person. Both sets can rightly be called sin.

Paul does not *always* use the word "flesh" of the sinful nature, however. The word is used quite flexibly by the apostle, although it generally connotes weakness and vulnerability. The fact that certain translations of the Bible render the word inconsistently (sometimes as "flesh," sometimes as "sinful nature," depending on context) is regrettable, obscuring the fact that both our moral weakness and our physical weakness are associated with the same thing, our flesh. Our flesh is weak.

Once we recognize this, we can begin to see how the overlapping problems associated with autism — on the one hand, anxiety and depression, and so on; on the other, addiction — might require a more integrated and embodied response, centering on our continuing constitutional weakness. It is not that one demands compassion while the other demands rebuke: both must be treated as outworking of our weakness and must be addressed in a redemptive way. Crucially, this forces us to recognize that the same essential reality is the hope that speaks to both: the presence of the Spirit of Jesus Christ with his people, in whom he is embodied. We must therefore approach all aspects of autism on the same terms, relating them to the reality of the incarnation of Jesus Christ, by which we are united to the life of God, a reality that is embodied within the church. If we lose sight of any of these elements, we will fail to deal rightly with the challenges of autism. Sin and suffering both need to be related to the gospel of Jesus Christ.

The integration of the two requires a properly developed theology of weakness.[20] In 2 Corinthians 3–4, Paul speaks of physically weak believers as the vessels in which the glory of God dwells. He represents their weakness, moreover, as necessary to the manifestation of that glory to the world. It is not just an unfortunate thing that God finds a way to work around: it is the medium *in* and *through* which his own strength is manifested.

> And all of us, with unveiled faces, seeing the glory of the Lord as though reflected in a mirror, are being transformed into the same image from one degree of glory to another; for this comes from the Lord, the Spirit. . . . (2 Cor 3:18)

⁶ For it is the God who said, "Let light shine out of darkness," who has shone in our hearts to give the light of the knowledge of the glory of God in the face of Jesus Christ.

⁷ But we have this treasure in clay jars, so that it may be made clear that this extraordinary power belongs to God and does not come from us. ⁸ We are afflicted in every way, but not crushed; perplexed, but not driven to despair; ⁹ persecuted, but not forsaken; struck down, but not destroyed; ¹⁰ always carrying in the body the death of Jesus, so that the life of Jesus may also be made visible in our bodies. ¹¹ For while we live, we are always being given up to death for Jesus' sake, so that the life of Jesus may be made visible in our mortal flesh. ¹² So death is at work in us, but life in you. (2 Cor 4:6-12)

This is part of a wider comparison that Paul develops between Moses, as the mediator of the old covenant, and both Jesus and believers, within the context of the new covenant.²¹ For this, he draws upon Exodus 34:30-35.

³⁰ When Aaron and all the Israelites saw Moses, the skin of his face was shining, and they were afraid to come near him. ³¹ But Moses called to them; and Aaron and all the leaders of the congregation returned to him, and Moses spoke with them. ³² Afterward all the Israelites came near, and he gave them in commandment all that the LORD had spoken with him on Mount Sinai. ³³ When Moses had finished speaking with them, he put a veil on his face; ³⁴ but whenever Moses went in before the LORD to speak with him, he would take the veil off, until he came out; and when he came out, and told the Israel-ites what he had been commanded, ³⁵ the Israelites would see the face of Moses, that the skin of his face was shining; and Moses would put the veil on his face again, until he went in to speak with him. (Exod 34:30-35)

Paul understands this story to indicate that Moses' radiance, which is a transmission of God's glory rather than a property native to him, is only ever unveiled for short periods as the law is communicated and is replenished as he spends time speaking

to God face to face. After he has communicated the commandments, shared the Torah, his face is veiled again. Paul's interpretation of this is that his face was veiled "to keep the people
of Israel from gazing at the end of the glory that was being set
aside" (2 Cor 2:13), an expression that points to the imperma-
nent glory of the old covenant. Paul initially compares the faces
of Moses and Jesus: where Moses provided limited access to the
glory, God has now shone in our hearts to give us the light of the
knowledge of God in the face of Jesus. But he not engaging in a
simple Jesus-Moses typology; his comparison is more pointedly
about the correspondences and differences between Moses and
Christian believers:

> [18] And all of us, with unveiled faces, seeing the glory of the
> Lord as though reflected in a mirror, are being transformed
> (metamorphosed) into the same image from one degree of
> glory to another; for this comes from the Lord, the Spirit.
> (2 Cor 3:18)

Moses' transformation was a temporary and unstable one, but
ours is a true and permanent one. This is linked to the imme-
diacy and fullness of the knowledge of God, who is directly
revealed to us in the face of Jesus Christ, but also to the reality
of the Spirit's work: "for this comes from the Lord, the Spirit."

Paul's use of the expression "and all of us" (*hēmeis de pantes*)
has a radically democratizing effect on this imagery. Despite the
fact that he is one of the few who has actually seen the face of
the glorified Jesus, something that seems to have had a dramatic
effect on his theology,[22] Paul is insistent that *all* believers have a
corresponding experience of God's glory, made real by the presence of the Spirit.

This brings us to our key point. The assertion that all believers reflect the glory of the Lord with unveiled faces would
appear to be at odds with the reality of our lives, at least as this
reality is perceived through sensory data: we remain lumps of

fragile flesh, subject to the weaknesses of our body, sometimes manifesting themselves in our mortality, sometimes in our sin. No one looking at us would see the glory that Paul has claimed we enjoy. Instead they would see weak, unimpressive, broken people. What is striking is that Paul does not move here to a crude dualism that affirms the spiritual and ignores the physical; rather, he emphasizes the necessity of our participation in the glory of God continuing to be experienced *through* our constitutional weakness. The image of treasure being contained in clay jars is triply suggestive: it signifies that the treasure is, to some extent, hidden, while also pointing to the ordinariness of that which it is hidden in. But it also suggests that the ordinariness is fragile: jars of clay are easily broken.[23]

It is striking, then, that Paul reaches the climax of his series of statements about the enduring of suffering by stating that we are "always carrying in the body the death of Jesus, *so that* the life of Jesus may also be made visible in our bodies" (2 Cor 4:10). In the following verse, he will reiterate this point, but now using our key word, "flesh." When read in conjunction with Galatians 2:20 ("the life I now live in the flesh I live by faith in the Son of God, who loved me and gave himself for me"), these verses point to the truth that our experience of salvation is not disembodied, but is lived within the context of the frailty of our flesh, which is both morally and physically needy. The God who gives life and light makes himself present with the flesh that can only live and grow by his indwelling presence, realized by the Spirit. Because he dwells in us, we can be "afflicted in every way, but not crushed; perplexed, but not driven to despair; persecuted, but not forsaken; struck down, but not destroyed" (2 Cor 4:8-9). Because his Spirit dwells in us, it is not inevitable that we will sin.

It is important to dwell for a moment on what Paul means when he speaks of our carrying "around in our body the death of Jesus" (2 Cor 4:10, NIV). It is easy to attenuate the significance of this, either to something *merely* mimetic, where we suffer in Christlike ways, or to something *merely* physical. If we approach it as something genuinely participatory, however, in which we truly *share* in the death of Jesus, then its significance can be seen as something radically more holistic. Such a reading is, I would suggest, demanded by the plain sense of Paul's words. He does not say, "we carry around something *like* the death of Jesus," but actually identifies what we carry *as* that death. This should be unsurprising, since elsewhere he speaks of those who have been baptized as being "united" to the death of Jesus (Rom 6:3-5). This is not simply substitutional language. Such language can be found elsewhere, but it is not what we see here. Instead, this is participatory language: we are in Christ, and have been united to his death, which we carry around in our bodies so that his life might also be visible.

I dwell on this because the Gospels show us moments when the embodied human mind of Jesus was overwhelmed, pressed down, and perplexed, and this is part of the reality in which we participate. In Gethsemane, he pleads for the cup to be taken away from him, yet does so in a way that submits to the will of God (Mark 14:32-42 and parallels). Luke recounts the same incident as one in which Jesus is in anguish (*agonia*), with his sweat "like great drops of blood falling down on the ground" (Luke 22:44). On the cross, he has no subjective sense of the presence of God the Father, and resorts to the words of Psalm 22: "My God, my God, why have you forsaken me?" Our accounts of atonement often explain away the true force of these words, sometimes in ways that are theologically problematic at the deepest of levels.[24] But we must allow their force to stand, and to speak to our interpretation of Paul's words in 2 Corinthians 4. When he speaks of the embodied struggle of the believer, he speaks of someone who is united to the sufferings of Christ, someone who may share in Christ's plea "take this cup from me"

or his cry "Why have you forsaken me?" The one who participates in the death and life of Jesus may share in his subjective anxiety, his subjective sense of bewilderment, even while
searching for the light that makes its way through the cracks.

This embodiment of our union with Christ is also, in important ways, corporate. Again, we noted in chapter 3 that Paul
sees the gospel manifesting itself among the body of Christ, the
church, the members of which are jointly united to him and to
each other. The image of the church as body is linked, for Paul,
to another corporate image, that of the temple whose corner-
stone is Christ. This same image is taken up by Peter, in ways
that are suggestive of suffering.

> [4] Coming to him, a living stone, rejected on one hand by mor-
> tals yet, to God on the other hand, chosen and precious, [5] as
> living stones you also are being built into a spiritual house, to
> be a holy priesthood to offer spiritual sacrifices acceptable to
> God through Jesus Christ. (1 Pet 2:4-5, my translation)

What is so important about this is that Peter identifies Jesus
as the living stone who has been rejected by men but chosen
by God and then applies this same identification to those being
built into the temple as they come to him—they, too, are living
stones. He continues to develop this imagery by quoting several
texts that share the imagery of stones, including Psalm 118:22
and Isaiah 28:16. The passage develops an important theme in
1 Peter, which is that the church united to Christ suffers with
him, and that its suffering, like his, is redemptively important
(cf. 1 Pet 1:3-9): it is not incidental to our participation in Christ,
but is part of our sharing in his kingdom and its growth.

All of this demands that we locate the suffering of the individual Christian within the body of Christ and recognize that
our experience of Christ's life is always embodied in this way.
The body must care for the suffering that afflicts any of its
members, but must do so in a way that seeks to make the life

of Christ in his Spirit the true source, not just of healing, but of the life that transfigures the weakness of our flesh. As we will see below, this requires a real care for the needs of those whose autism brings genuine suffering and distress, to them and to those around them.

"The Flesh," Sin, and Addiction

We need to reflect further on why the same word, "flesh," is used by Paul in relation to our constitutional sinfulness. The word, as we have just noted, does not *necessarily* indicate sinfulness, and at points it can be used positively of the human nature of Jesus (cf. Rom 1:3 and 9:5). Predominantly, however, Paul does use it in a way that is particularly oriented toward our constitutional sinfulness. How do we explain this range of uses, and how might it be brought to bear on our doctrine of sin?

The concept that binds the uses is probably that of weakness, conceived in terms of helplessness. Flesh was created to be in fellowship with the life of God; isolated from that life or taken in itself, it lacks all life, potency, and goodness. Its impotence to flourish in any way, either physically or morally, makes it vulnerable to participation in the reality of sin, something that emerges in Paul's words:

> For I know that nothing good dwells within me, that is, in my flesh. I can will what is right, but I cannot do it. (Rom 7:18)

There is a real culpability that goes with this, as helpless flesh actively participates in evil. Pauline scholars tend to overlook some of the background to Paul's language of the flesh, which is found in the flood account of Genesis. There the problem is that flesh has filled the world with violence:

> [12] And God saw that the earth was corrupt; for all flesh had corrupted its ways upon the earth. [13] And God said to Noah, "I have determined to make an end of all flesh, for the earth

is filled with violence because of them; now I am going to destroy them along with the earth." (Gen 6:12-13)

The helplessness of flesh does not lead to a moral inertia, but to a pursuit of the wrong things, a plunging into violence. Of course, Noah becomes a locus for divine grace and the flood story becomes one of restoration, rather than merely destruction. But it contributes to a biblical account of embodied human life that sees flesh, when separated from the life of God, as helpless to flourish and hence bound to sin. This also explains why the same transformational presence that fills our frail bodies with divine life is represented as the key to overcoming this condition of moral helplessness:

> Instead, put on the Lord Jesus Christ, and make no provision for the flesh, to gratify its desires. (Rom 13:14)

The answer to the weakness of flesh is never anything other than the personal presence of Jesus Christ, realized in the presence of his Spirit.

> [3] For God has done what the law, weakened by the flesh, could not do: by sending his own Son in the likeness of sinful flesh, and to deal with sin, he condemned sin in the flesh, [4] so that the just requirement of the law might be fulfilled in us, who walk not according to the flesh but according to the Spirit. (Rom 8:3-4)

As we saw in the previous section, this is not a dualism in which the flesh is left behind or discounted, but rather one in which it is no longer powerless and hence subject to its own enslavement. Just as our weak flesh now becomes the context in which the glory of Christ is embodied, so it becomes the context in which the goodness of Christ is manifest. That goodness is realized within us by the Spirit:

[16] Live by the Spirit, I say, and do not gratify the desires of the flesh. [17] For what the flesh desires is opposed to the Spirit, and what the Spirit desires is opposed to the flesh; for these are opposed to each other, to prevent you from doing what you want. (Gal 5:16-17)

Paul's eventual hope for the Christian life is one that involves a transformation, as the body is finally and fully transformed by the presence of the Spirit. This is the core of the teaching on resurrection in 1 Corinthians 15, where Paul speaks of our final state as involving a "spiritual" body (1 Cor 15:44). His teaching is set as the answer to the question "How are the dead raised? With what kind of body do they come?" He is careful to stress that we will indeed have bodies, but affirms this in a way that recognizes that bodies and species are different:

[39] Not all flesh is alike, but there is one flesh for human beings, another for animals, another for birds, and another for fish. [40] There are both heavenly bodies and earthly bodies, but the glory of the heavenly is one thing, and that of the earthly is another. . . .

[42] So it is with the resurrection of the dead. What is sown is perishable, what is raised is imperishable. [44] . . . It is sown a physical body, it is raised a spiritual body (1 Cor 15:39-40, 42, 44a)

When he speaks of the spiritual body, then, he identifies it as a particular *kind* of body, a distinctive *kind* of flesh. The spiritual body remains a corporeal one.

But what does it mean for this body to be "spiritual"? The adjective that Paul uses is *pneumatikos*. As Gordon Fee noted in his classic study of Paul's teaching on the Holy Spirit, *God's Empowering Presence*,[25] the meaning of any adjective is linked to the usage of the cognate noun. When a gardener uses the word "dirty," for example, we expect it to have a meaning that is defined by a largely positive experience of dirt; when a journalist uses the same word, drawing on a different association of the word "dirt" (as something that might be "dished"), the meaning will likely be more negative. Of course, the gardener might hurl it as an expletive while reading a newspaper, and the journalist might spend an afternoon in their own garden. But the context will generally make clear how the word is being used, what it is associated with.

The point of note here is that Paul has predominantly used the noun "spirit" (*pneuma*) in 1 Corinthians of God's Spirit and has, indeed, repeatedly identified that Spirit with the one God of the Shema and his one mediator, Jesus Christ:

> For in the one Spirit we were all baptized into one body—Jews or Greeks, slaves or free—and we were all made to drink of one Spirit. (1 Cor 12:13; cf. 8:6)

When we come to 2 Corinthians, this association is developed further with the remarkable identification of the Spirit in 3:18, "This comes from the Lord, the Spirit." Predominantly, then, within the Corinthian correspondence, Paul uses the word *pneuma* in relation to the Holy Spirit, who appears to be identified with God in rather personal terms. If we turn to Romans 8, we have an extensive account of how the Spirit works within us, which is quite striking in its representation of the Spirit as a person who dwells (8:9, 11) and who is the co-subject of the verbs that speak of Christian life: the Spirit co-testifies with our spirit that we are the children of God. This is an interesting example, for it affirms the place of the individual Christian's spirit, but in the context of a passage that is predominantly concerned with the Holy Spirit.

A more extensive theological account of the Spirit would consider the material in the Synoptic Gospels and in John, where the Spirit is identified in personal terms, but we can allow this brief survey of some of Paul's material to speak to his use of the adjective "spiritual" in 1 Corinthians 15. Given his predominant use of *pneuma* to refer to the Holy Spirit, especially within 1 Corinthians, it is most likely that the *pneumatikos* body is one that derives its character from the Holy Spirit. Such an interpretation is at odds with approaches that have understood the expression principally against a Stoic background,[26] but make good sense of Paul's emphasis on the place of the Holy Spirit as the defining marker of the believer's life. It also makes good sense of why he describes the current experience of the Spirit as "first fruits" that anticipate the full redemption of our bodies (Rom 8:23) or a "down payment" (*arrabōn*, 2 Cor 1:22, my translation): the new covenant is the covenant of the Spirit (2 Cor 3:6) and will reach its fulfillment when our bodies become Spirit-bodies in the fullest sense.

Taken together with the previous section, this provides us with some important groundwork for our reflections upon how the weakness of our flesh, manifest in the co-occurrence of other conditions with autism, might be accommodated, addressed, and cared for lovingly within the church, the body of Christ. By the Spirit, we can put to death the acts of the flesh. It will not happen immediately, and does not bypass our own agency, as co-subjects of the acts associated with the Spirit's work in us: we must seek to be led by the Spirit and helped by him. It will also not happen in isolation: the Spirit works in and through the members of the body of Christ. As much as we might prefer to be alone, and to pursue our vocation alone, we are incorporated into the body of Christ and placed in transformational fellowship with its members.

Embodied Salvation

Redeemed Flesh and the Community of Christ

We have seen the consistent emphasis on the embodiment of the gospel as involving the body of Christ, the community of the church. Now we must begin to apply what we have seen throughout this chapter to how the members of the body show love toward those in their midst with autism, and their families or caregivers, particularly as they experience the genuine difficulties that we have discussed here.

The first point is simply to stress the obligation of those in the body of Christ to approach the difficult behaviors of its members through the gospel and in light of its truth. Those who are depressed or anxious and those who are addicted to substances or activities do not cease to be members of the body of Christ: the ultimate significance of their actions is determined by the gospel and cannot, in the end, undo the gospel. We are obligated to deal with each other in love and to deal with the weaknesses of others with compassion. This, of course, should be a basic value among those who are united to Jesus, the head of the body, who is also its high priest, "able to deal gently with the ignorant and wayward, since he himself is subject to weakness" (Heb 5:2).

In this regard, it is important to note the positioning of Paul's famous discourse on the character of love in 1 Corinthians 13. It comes immediately after his extensive teaching on the oneness of the body and the obligation of its members to care for each other (1 Cor 12), which itself follows his teaching on the unity that is demanded by the Lord's Supper (1 Cor 11), in turn embedded within a part of the letter explicitly controlled by the implications of the Shema: the Lord is one, with one mediator and one Spirit from which we have all been made to drink. The one body united to him eats from one loaf and is required to manifest his unity within itself, particularly as it deals with the weakness of its members. When this is brought to 1 Corinthians 13, the implications for how Christians must deal with the difficult behaviors of other members of the body of Christ should be clear:

> [4] Love is patient; love is kind; love is not envious or boastful or arrogant [5] or rude. It does not insist on its own way; it is not irritable or resentful; [6] it does not rejoice in wrongdoing, but

rejoices in the truth. [7] It bears all things, believes all things, hopes all things, endures all things. (1 Cor 13:4-7)

Many autistic individuals, or their families, will testify that fellow Christians have failed to bear all things or endure all things, and have not been kind. This is something of which we must repent.

Second, the members of the body must recognize their obligation to address the ways in which they have contributed to the problems. As we have seen, while comorbidities may be traced to underlying physical or neurophysiological factors that are not easily treated, they are also often compounded or triggered by environmental factors that can more easily be addressed. Anxiety and depression may be triggered or exacerbated by the social and sensory environment of the world, including the particular ways in which the world is instantiated in the church. Social and sensory elements do not cause the anxiety or depression, it is important to note; the actual cause is deeper. This means that we cannot ascribe blame to those who have unwittingly intensified the anxiety of a person with autism by whistling, wearing deodorant, failing to operate the PA system properly, or insisting on a conversation. But we can expect them to do something about it once they know that it has a destructive effect. This is why autism awareness is so important within the church: we need to learn to accommodate the sensory and social needs of those within the church, and to be aware that the effects of failing to accommodate them can be really terrible.

Third, the members of the body must seek to help each other, sometimes by consolation and sometimes by challenge. We allow the word of Christ to dwell in us as we teach and admonish each other, singing in psalms, hymns, and spiritual songs (Col 3:16). We strengthen weak limbs "so that the lame may not fall by the wayside, but be healed" (Heb 12:13, my translation).[27]

Formation, Adaptation, and Gratitude

For autistic people, and those who may care for them, it is particularly important to recognize the possibility of change and some of the ways that this is represented in the Bible. Change is typically more difficult for those with autism, but it is not impossible. Within the clinical literature, the term that is often used is "adaptation." More and more research has emerged in recent years that demonstrates the possibility of successful adaptation in autistic persons, particularly children, when appropriate educational interventions are made. In the case of children, a set of strategies has been developed that makes use of LEGO.[28] There is also a growing body of testimony about the effects of mindfulness training and meditation, which is interesting not least because there is also a good deal of evidence for the efficacy of these in treating addictive behaviors and anxiety. All of this is connected to a general shift in medical literature toward recognizing the plasticity of the brain throughout life and its capacity to adapt.

It is important to distinguish "adaptation" from "camouflaging," which merely masks a problem by superficially imitating the behaviors of others in order to fit in to their expectations. It does not really address the problem and may, in certain cases, compound it, particularly when the behaviors imitated are actually quite bad in themselves. As we noted in chapter 1, many autistic people are quite skilled at camouflaging, which is one of the reasons that the incidence of autism within the female population has been underestimated until recently.

True adaptation involves more than just masking behaviors in order to fit in; it involves addressing the things that keep us from flourishing. The traditional educational language that was used to describe this was that of "formation," a term that has been taken into the theological traditions and used effectively in relation to Christian growth. Properly understood, the language of formation can be usefully brought into the conversation about autism. Formation recognizes that our capacity to flourish is limited or compromised by the disordered character of our instincts and passions; the path to flourishing opens when we gain control of those instincts by ordering them properly, under the regulation of our mind. This kind of language has an obvious appeal to autistic people, who tend to like order, particularly where it is governed by the mind.[29]

This is the classical grounding for all concepts of virtue: the virtuous person is one who has learned to order themselves well and, in doing so, is capable of accomplishing greater things than they could previously. When brought into Christian theology, of course, the concept of virtuous formation must be modified to take into account what is said about sin and about Christ: sin is so deep in our constitution that we cannot tame it ourselves, but only in union with Christ and his Spirit. Moreover, the goal of our flourishing is not to become better versions of ourselves, as in classical virtue theory, but to inhabit and embody the moral identity of Christ, to become radically different persons.[30] For persons with autism, this may be a particularly difficult concept to envision, but it cannot be bypassed without distorting the gospel.

There is a good deal that can be appropriated from the formational traditions and from the contemporary resurgence of interest in them among psychologists and counselors.[31] Here I want to focus on two elements that are particularly prominent in the New Testament representations of formational growth and how they might bear on addiction, anxiety, and depression.

The first element is that it is storied. The stories that we read shape us and rewire our brains; there is evidence that reading certain books affects our cognition differently than reading other books. The person who reads the Harry Potter books will know the world differently than the one who reads *Twilight*, and differently than the one who reads both.[32] All accounts of Christian formation necessarily draw the believer to read and to reflect

upon the fourfold gospel narratives of Jesus Christ, set within
the stories of God's dealings with the world, as their story. This
is actually a much denser and more complex statement than it
might appear at first. To read the gospel stories is to recognize
that *those* events are the truly pivotal ones for *us*, relativizing the
importance of the immediate realities of our current experience.
Those events are pivotal because of the identity of the one who
is at the heart of those events: his experience and his character, realized within the story, determine the truths of history on
either side of them, conditioning God's relationship to the entire
cosmos from before time began and into eternity. They condition
and determine his relationship to us, to me, whatever my most
recent sin or most recent reiteration of my addiction might look
like. This speaks to my anxiety; it gives hope in the darkness.

And, as we read of his self-sacrifice, and the mastery of his
anxieties that was required, the pattern of his behavior can be
mapped into our own neurology. Our minds can be renewed
(Rom 12:2) as we are transformed into the likeness of the one
to whom we are united by the Spirit who brings freedom (2 Cor
3:18). This is not just imitation, but something more profound,
linked at once to our recognition that his story has become *our*
story and to the acknowledgment that the presence of the Spirit
makes this more than just wordplay—he makes it reality.

Jesus is not the only character, however, with whom we
identify in our reading of the Gospels. He is surrounded by a
group of disciples who, for readers, seem frustratingly blind
to the truth and incompetent as followers. That changes in the
book of Acts, as the Spirit transforms them, but it remains the
case that we have a complex of identifications at work in our
readings of the gospel, not just with Jesus but with his disciples; not just with the hero (if that is indeed the right word)[33]
but with a group of followers who are not quite villains, but are
also not quite ideal. If our stories are absorbed into the story of

Jesus, just as theirs were, we are led to expect something other than triumphalism, but that nevertheless represents real change, wrought in us by Christ's Spirit.[34]

At this point, I would expect—and even hope—that readers of this book will observe that this assumes that the Christian with autism can read, which is not true for every autistic person. In fact, through the history of the church, *most* Christians have been illiterate; high levels of literacy are a largely modern phenomenon, and even then are confined to particular cultural or geographical areas. The gospel was *heard*, usually in the context of liturgy, and may also have been *seen* in artistic or iconic depictions. What this highlights for us is the importance of reading the Bible to those who cannot read it for themselves, whether because they have limited literacy or are entirely nonverbal. We will say more about nonverbal autism in the next chapter. Here we can simply note that reading the Bible in the hearing of those who cannot read it for themselves opens possibilities that we may never be able to understand or investigate for God to work through his word in their lives.

The second element that must be highlighted is the place of prayerful gratitude in the life of the believer. Gratitude has become an important element in popular psychology, helping those who practice it to appreciate the world beyond themselves and thereby to find happiness. Immanuel Kant famously saw ingratitude—along with several other deficiencies—as the essence of vileness,[35] and the recent interest in gratitude acknowledges that its recovery can be an important part of human flourishing.

For Christians, gratitude is an important part of prayer. It serves as more than just a practice by which we enumerate the good things that have happened to us (although that is something important in its own right). More importantly, it serves as an act by which we acknowledge that we inhabit a divine economy that is defined by the grace and goodness of God. At the heart of so much that is difficult in the experience of autism is the need to find some kind of control over the world in which we live. Gratitude acknowledges that such control will always be limited, because the true lordship of all things lies with God, who is the providential ruler of all things and the one who gives his life into all things.

To practice gratitude is not necessarily an easy thing, and it can be more difficult in some regards for those who are autistic. To learn to trust in the God to whom we are grateful, likewise, is not an easy thing. But interestingly, the more we practice gratitude, the more we uncurve from ourselves and open ourselves to those to whom we are grateful;[36] the more we practice gratitude, the easier gratitude becomes. And the easier gratitude becomes, the easier trust becomes. It is striking, then, that Paul writes to the Philippians:

> [6] Do not worry about anything, but in everything by prayer and supplication with thanksgiving let your requests be made known to God. [7] And the peace of God, which surpasses all understanding, will guard your hearts and your minds in Christ Jesus. (Phil 4:6-7)

Paul's language assumes that there are triggers for anxiety; he does not deny the reality of these. He directs his readers to bring these triggers to God in prayer and supplication, but with thanksgiving. The peace of God that accompanies such prayerful gratitude protects the heart and mind, the very parts of us that are so vulnerable to anxiety and depression and that often seek to deal with these by repeating familiar behaviors. That peace cannot entirely be explained or described; it "surpasses all understanding," but it can be experienced, even by those of us who are constitutionally vulnerable to distress.

Another passage in the New Testament speaks to this. Jesus promises rest to those who are weary and heavy laden (Matt

11:28-30). Immediately before this, he has given thanks to the Father that he has hidden truths from the wise and revealed them to infants, through his own role as the Son who reveals the Father. It is a fascinating passage, on one level because it challenges our continuing tendency to value the socially and intellectually impressive over those who are undeveloped, like children; this is surely relevant in relation to those with autism whose development is compromised.[37] On another level, it is fascinating because it presents the one through whom we have access to God as himself the embodiment of gratitude. We come to one who is grateful, and it is in his gratitude to the Father that he gives us rest. When we bring this together with the recognition that our lives are absorbed into the story of Jesus Christ as rendered to us in the Bible, it has a remarkable capacity to lead us to inhabit the kind of gratitude that can bring us peace.

Conclusions

This has been a difficult chapter to write and may have been a difficult chapter to read, for it has forced us to consider the reality of the challenges that can come with autism. It is a condition that can be accompanied by depression and anxiety, and by destructive addictions. These are real forms of suffering that can involve real evil and real guilt.

We must always approach such issues in the context of the gospel. The basis of our hope is Jesus Christ, his person and work, realized in us through the Spirit. His potency is the key truth upon which our hope is founded, not our own faithfulness or experience. We trust that this reality will manifest itself in our lives in transformational ways, but our faith is always defined by its object, not by our character as believers. This is true for those who deal pastorally with the difficult realities that accompany autism, and it is true for those who are autistic believers, as they seek to relate their faith properly to their painful experiences.

Our weakness is not the definitive reality: it is always located within a bigger account of God's determination to see us flourish.

The problems that we deal with all emerge from the weakness of our constitution, our flesh. We saw that for Paul this weakness is sometimes moral and sometimes physical, but the answer to this weakness is always the life-giving presence of God, brought to us with gentleness by Jesus Christ. This does not minimize the importance of our own participation in this reality, as we pursue formation through the work of Christ's Spirit in the body of the church. It grounds our hope that as we read Scripture, pursue self-discipline, and minister to each other, we will see real change as God works in us. Our hope, as believers, is that this present reality that we experience is not all that there is and all that there ever will be. In Christ, by the Spirit, we can be transformed and renewed.

6

AUTISM AND CHRISTIAN PRACTICES
The Challenge of Pastoral Care

This chapter is something of a miscellany. In it, I will think about several different experiences that have repeatedly been described by autistic people or their families and caregivers as they negotiate what it means to be a Christian with autism. Some of these involve distinctive challenges that are not universally experienced by persons with autism—it is a spectrum, after all—but are described frequently enough to warrant some discussion here. Others simply involve different ways of processing the core practices of Christian faith, such as reading the Bible. My intention throughout is to highlight parts of the Bible that might speak to the challenges, or practices of reading the Bible that might allow a different way of thinking about them. Underpinning all of this is a recognition of what is sometimes referred to as "the tyranny of the normal": once certain things are considered to be "normal," other practices or experience tend to be labeled as "abnormal." We need to recognize that this can cause us to undervalue or even reject experiences and practices that may not be typical, but that may nevertheless be valid realities within God's providential dealing with his creatures. I have here used the word "providential," deliberately invoking the discussion of providence in chapter 3, where we highlighted that the doctrine allows us to speak of the distinctive telos of each individual creature and the distinctive way in which God relates intimately to them. In this chapter, we will consider some specific examples of such providential particularity.

The experiences and challenges I describe in this chapter have not, for the most part, emerged from my research as such. They have not been described in answers to carefully designed qualitative analysis questions. They have instead emerged from friendships and from the conversations that naturally take place within them, as parents of children with autism and friends who have been diagnosed (or who await a diagnosis) share some of their experience, including their anxieties. My own research is into the biblical material, not into these conversations; they have simply prompted me to ask a particular set of questions that might not have occurred to me otherwise.

If You (Cannot) Confess with Your Lips That Jesus Is Lord

Profound Autism and the Impossible Profession of Faith

Some autistic persons are profoundly affected by the condition, to the point where they are either nonverbal or minimally verbal. This is not the same as saying that they cannot communicate: communication does not have to involve words, and shared actions may allow the person with autism to communicate something to those around them, even if this act of communication leaves open a great deal of space for interpretation. Rowan Williams, in his theological study of language *The Edge of Words*, devotes a chapter to reflecting on how such acts of communication may be significant.[1] While there may be communication of a certain kind, however, there will never be a capacity for verbal speech in some persons with autism, even the kind of verbal speech that might be articulated in formal sign language.

Parents of children with autism who are minimally verbal are often anxious at some level about whether their children can properly fulfill what is required to become a Christian, since they will never be able to confess with their lips that "Jesus is Lord" (Rom 10:9; cf. 1 Cor 12:3). Since this kind of autism also involves cognitive difficulties, this concern can be linked to the question of whether they also fulfill the other part of the expectation in Romans 10:9, believing in their heart that God raised Jesus from the dead. I noted that this anxiety operates "at some level": in truth, most Christian parents have a general sense that God will work differently in the life of their child, accommodating their difficulties, and trust in this truth. But some anxieties can remain, and my intention here is to reflect on how we can read the Bible in a way that speaks to them.

Let me share an insight from a conversation with a friend of mine, my former pastor who semiretired to the Western Isles of Scotland, where he worked with a congregation in the Free Church of Scotland. He found that despite the relatively high number of people involved in the church who have profound developmental disabilities, this anxiety is largely absent among Christians there. They are quite confident that those who cannot say "Jesus is Lord" with their lips can be Christians. His own sense was that this reflected a strong theology of regeneration in Scottish Calvinist theology: faith and confession are simply the expressions of God's transforming and recreative work within us. They are *normally* vital to the Christian life, but not because they fulfill conditions as "works"; rather, it is because they are the appropriate responses to God's prior activity.

This, I think, provides a helpful inroad into thinking about the biblical material, particularly when we take seriously the truth that God will deal with his people in providentially particular ways. It calls attention to examples within Scripture where we see responses to God's work made by those whose cognitive development will not allow them to inhabit a position of faith than can be articulated in propositions ("Jesus is Lord"; "God raised him from the dead") and whose physical development does not allow them to utter words with their lips.

One example of this is the unborn John the Baptist, who leaps for joy in his mother's womb at the sound of Mary's greeting (Luke 1:41, 44). Here, of course, we are speaking about a child at a particular stage of development, who will in due course grow to maturity with a normally functional set of cognitive faculties, if with an unusual dress sense. The point, though, is that even in his fetal condition he is capable of responding in an appropriate way to the presence of his unborn Savior. His faculties are not yet capable of processing propositions or holding beliefs, his brain is not yet able to cognitively process sensory experiences in ways that are intelligible, and yet he is able to respond to the manifestation of God's grace in the only way he can, by kicking his little heart out.

We can ask about John's own subsequent development — including his questioning of whether Jesus was the Messiah and the way that he is represented as the last of the old covenant prophets, whose status is exceeded by the least in the kingdom of heaven (Luke 7:20-28; Matt 11:2-15) — but this should not detract from the way that Luke's narrative represents his response to Jesus as a manifestation of the Spirit's presence within him (cf. Luke 1:15).

This example allows us to approach Romans 8:26 and its wider context as a further example of nonverbal communication. Here, Paul speaks of the Spirit interceding for the one who is not able to pray with "groans that words cannot express" (Rom 8:26, NIV, 1984 ed.). The Greek here is somewhat difficult to interpret and requires a little depth of study. Because it is an important passage, I will reproduce the text in Greek and in transliteration before offering my own translation of it.

> [26] Ὡσαύτως δὲ καὶ τὸ πνεῦμα συναντιλαμβάνεται τῇ ἀσθενείᾳ ἡμῶν· τὸ γὰρ τί προσευξώμεθα καθὸ δεῖ οὐκ οἴδαμεν, ἀλλὰ αὐτὸ τὸ πνεῦμα ὑπερεντυγχάνει στεναγμοῖς ἀλαλήτοις· [27] ὁ δὲ ἐραυνῶν τὰς καρδίας οἶδεν τί τὸ φρόνημα τοῦ πνεύματος, ὅτι κατὰ θεὸν ἐντυγχάνει ὑπὲρ ἁγίων.

> [26] *Hōsautōs de kai to pneuma synantilambanetai tē astheneia hēmōn; to gar ti proseuxōmetha katho dei ouk oidamen, alla auto to pneuma hyperentygchanei stenagmois alalētois;* [27] *ho de eraunōn tas kardias oiden ti to phronēma tou pneumatos, hoti kata theon entygchanei hyper hagiōn.*

> [26] Likewise, the Spirit co-assists (or "helps") us in our weakness; for we do not know what we ought to pray, but that same Spirit intercedes with groans that cannot be articulated in words, [27] and the one who searches hearts knows the mind of the Spirit, for according to [the will of] God does he intercede for the saints. (Rom 8:26-27, my translation)

My translation is deliberately awkward because I want to call attention to several elements within the text. First, the word for "helps" (*synantilambanetai*, from *synatilambanō*) is a compound verb that includes the prefix *syn-*, which means "together with"; this is why I have rather stiffly translated the verb as "co-assists." The *syn-* prefix occurs frequently through Romans 8 to indicate the mutual activity of Christ and his Spirit with the spirit of the individual Christian. We are not the sole subjects of the verbs of activity that are used of the Christian life; we act with Christ and with the Spirit. Here, then, our act of prayer is represented as one in which the Spirit's agency works with ours, but does so particularly at a point where our minds do not have the capacity to identify appropriate language to render what we need to pray. The Spirit's intercession does not give us words at this point, but gives us groans that cannot be articulated in words (*stenagmois alalētois*). Some have understood this to indicate the practice of speaking in tongues, but the plain sense of the expression is that these groans are not acts of language; they are "unspeakable."[2] Interestingly, too, they involve a participation in the mind of God's Spirit that is beyond our own capacity to process cognitively: we "do not know" (*ouk oidamen*) what we ought to pray (literally, "what to pray as necessary"), but when God searches our hearts "he knows" (*oiden*) the mind of the Spirit (*to phronēma tou pneumatos*), since the Spirit intercedes according to the will of God. Literally, this is "according to God," but adding the words "the will of" makes sense of the construction.

Thus, the believer here does not themselves understand, in a cognitive sense, what they are doing or saying, but they participate in something bigger than themselves, as the Spirit works in them. We should note, too, the presence of the word that has repeatedly surfaced in this book, particularly when we read the writings of Paul: "weakness" (*astheneia*). This work of the Spirit allows those who are weak to share in the very mind of God, even as their own minds are overwhelmed by the reality of the situation. As I write, I am struck that this may be as relevant to the experience of meltdown as it is to the experience of the non-verbal autistic person in prayer.

Here again, we must note that we are not talking about the person with autism, but about something that can be seen to correspond to the phenomena experienced by those who are nonverbal or minimally verbal. The reality of our participation in the Spirit's work is not compromised by the absence of language, and, perhaps more importantly, neither is it compromised by our own limited cognitive grasp of what it is that we participate in. This leaves room for us to say that the *typical* experience of the Christian *will* be one involving language and understanding (if of a limited and creaturely kind), but that the normality of that experience does not negate the reality of other kinds of experience.

One last point might be added to our discussion of Romans 8. Paul seems deliberately to link the groans of the believers who await the redemption of their bodies to those of the creation as it eagerly awaits the freedom of the glory of the children of God (Rom 8:21-22). While we can consider this groaning to be metaphorical, and can reflect on what Paul might be thinking of (earthquakes, volcanic eruptions, etc.), the connections that Paul draws between the creation's expression of its response to God and ours is suggestive of providence. God is leading all things to their eventual purpose, and, as he does so, they respond. Their responses reflect what they are and what they can do: the earth cannot confess with its lips that Jesus is Lord, the mountains cannot believe in their hearts that God raised him. But their responses are meaningful nonetheless: as God leads the cosmos to its fulfillment, the creation groans, and the believer groans. They groan together, incapable of comprehending the work of God or articulating their place within it, but responding truly to the Spirit's work.

From this, we can return to Romans 10:9 with a new set of insights to frame how we read the text. An important initial observation concerning the passage as a whole is that Paul is concerned here to frame the act of proclamation: he is concerned to assert that the key thing for Israel is that they hear (or have heard) the message of the gospel.

[14] But how are they to call on one in whom they have not believed? And how are they to believe in one of whom they have never heard? And how are they to hear without someone to proclaim him? [15] And how are they to proclaim him unless they are sent? As it is written, "How beautiful are the feet of those who bring good news!" (Rom 10:14-15)

He goes on to discuss the question of whether Israel has already heard that message and what its reaction to it involved. The interpretation of the wider section of Romans (chapters 9–11) is notoriously controverted in biblical scholarship, but the core point for us is straightforward: when Paul speaks about confession and belief, it is not to establish a particular bar that one must clear in order to be considered an insider, but rather to contrast an account of salvation that centers on one's response to a message about something done *for us* to one that centers on something we do ourselves. Paul is actually concerned to show how open the way to salvation is, which is why the verses that follow 10:9 are so inclusive:

> [12] For there is no distinction between Jew and Greek; the same Lord is Lord of all and is generous to all who call on him. [13] For, "Everyone who calls on the name of the Lord shall be saved." (Rom 10:12-13)

Once this is recognized, we can see that Paul is concerned in the preceding verses to stress the availability of this message:

> But what does it say?
>   "The word is near you,
>   on your lips and in your heart"
> (that is, the word of faith that we proclaim). (Rom 10:8)

These words, and those that precede them, are taken from Deuteronomy 30:14 and its wider context, where the LORD makes clear to Israel that he has given them what they need and expects them to respond appropriately: they do not need to ascend into heaven or to cross to the other side of the sea to find some further revelation that will enable them to live morally successful lives. What they need is already near to them; it is on their lips and in their hearts. Paul takes up this language and maps it onto the gospel message: what is on our lips is the confession that Jesus is Lord, and what is in our hearts is the conviction that

God raised him from the dead. This is what we have in Romans 10:9. But the point of this is to stress the simplicity and availability of salvation: this word is near us, and we do not need to add to it our own works. Within the wider passage, however it is to be understood as a whole, Paul is clearly considering the particular question of how Israel has responded to this message.

When read in the light of Romans 8 and the story of the unborn John, these verses no longer seem to speak about a *sine qua non* practice necessary to salvation, but rather to describe the responsive character of Christian faith and the availability of the message to which this response is made. That recognition allows us to affirm that such a response may well look different for the person whose neurophysiological development is atypical, but that God in his providence can lead them to respond rightly to the presence of the word and of the Spirit of the word. For the parent, caregiver, or friend who deals with a nonverbal person with autism, whose communication is limited to wordless groaning, this insight may be profoundly important.

Prayer

Prayer is a central practice of Christian life, yet parents of children on the autism spectrum will often talk about the difficulty the children have with prayer. This can present a difficulty in conceiving a practice that is directed toward a person who is not physically present; communicating with people who are present can be challenging enough, and communicating with someone who is not can obviously pose further conceptual difficulties. A further difficulty can lie in verbally articulating needs that the person in question might not normally feel any obligation to share. If, as an autistic person, I do not tend to communicate easily what I am thinking or how I am feeling to the people around me, how can I easily do so with God? Finally, prayer is (like all interactive communication) an improvisational activity;

at least, this is the kind of prayer that poses difficulties for children with autism, and perhaps for adults.

This last point might suggest a helpful way to respond to the challenge. All improvisational skills are built through the practicing of patterns and the replication of forms learned from others. Musicians learn skills and scales in order to improvise, and their improvisations are often informed by patterns or movements that they have learned from others and now bend to their particular creative context. Improvisation in music is never a free-for-all; it can only really be done by those who have attained a certain degree of mastery. Something similar can be said for improvisational comedy or even improvisational preaching: those who are good at it typically draw upon a rich awareness of what will trigger certain reactions, through the deployment of certain kinds of wordplay (perhaps even a bank of jokes that can be modified to purpose) and with a certain communicative skill set. Again, brilliant improvisational comedians, like brilliant improvisational preachers or teachers, have often reached a certain level of mastery, often through the imitation of others.

The same parts of the brain that are involved in improvisational music are engaged in normal interactive conversation.[3] My friend and fellow New Testament scholar Constantine Campbell uses this to illustrate the fact that anyone can learn to engage in improvisational music if they can acquire the confidence to engage those parts of the brain that they would use when talking to a friend. Of course, even this kind of improvisational speech draws upon a childhood of acquiring language skills and vocabulary and a life of acquiring habits of speech and turns of phrase. How many of us have, at some point, thrown a line from a TV show, or even just a way of speaking that replicates a character, into our own improvisational speech? This can sometimes reflect our having shared cultural texts that bind persons of particular cultures and times. In the 1990s, expressions used by the characters in *Friends* became everyday speech; just as interestingly, the way that certain characters would intone certain words became characteristic of *everyone's* speech. All interactive speech—from chatting to interviewing—is constructed from building blocks shaped by imitation.

This is also true of prayer. There are undoubtedly cultures of prayer that characterize different traditions. In my background, prayers were usually formulated in the English of the King James Version Bible (using "thou," "thee," and "thy," for example) and would involve a particular set of nonbiblical expressions that were tacitly understood to characterize pious prayer. When I arrived at university, I encountered Christians who had very different cultures of prayer; they used "you" when addressing God and always seemed to preface their supplications with the word "just," as if to ensure that the request was appropriately modest. None of this is necessarily a bad thing; it simply illustrates that our improvisational prayers are constructed from elements that we have learned through our cultures, by the imitation of other Christians.

This kind of improvisation through imitation might be more challenging for those with autism (although they can often develop good mimicry skills), but it may also be possible to acquire it through the right kind of study, with a little extra work. Even if not, there may be other kinds of prayer than the improvisational sort, and these may be especially important for those with autism.

The Bible itself contains prayers, which both model prayer and function as prayers that believers can read and make their own. Jesus, of course, was approached by his disciples with a request that he teach them how to pray (Luke 11:1); the "Lord's Prayer" that he taught them is often seen as a model for how prayer should be structured, but it is also a prayer that is widely read as a core Christian practice. The words with which Jesus introduces the prayer ("When you pray, say . . .": Luke 11:2; "Pray, therefore, like this . . .": Matt 6:9; translations mine) indicate that this is a prayer that is to be repeated, not just imitated. In the New Testament, we also have various prayers of Paul recorded for us, which might also function as prayers that can be read by believers as their own prayer.

Most strikingly, we have the book of Psalms. The psalms are songs, but they are also prayers. Interestingly, through the history of the church, whenever the gospel has moved into a new linguistic territory, the psalms are often the first thing to be translated after the four Gospels. This should be unsurprising to us, because the psalms really constitute the Bible's own prayer book. And it is a prayer book that covers the range of emotional and psychological challenges encountered by believers. To read through the psalms is to read through a remarkable collection of prayers that are willing to express hope and confidence, but also shame, anger, anguish, and fear; the psalmists are prepared to voice their ugliest instincts to God and to appear before him in whatever condition they find themselves. This means we need to be careful when reading the psalms, but it also makes this book of prayers into a remarkable resource for the Christian. They can empower us to pray things that we would not have the confidence to say otherwise ("How long, O LORD? Will you hide yourself forever?": Ps 89:46). Of course, they were written long before the time of Jesus, and this needs to be factored into *how* we read them as Christians, but this is not a reason to marginalize them from our life of prayer and reading.

Practically, the psalms give us a prayer book that we can work through and read out as our own prayers. I have often found that when trying to engage with the psalms simply as readings, the resonance between the psalmists' words and circumstances and my own has led to them spontaneously becoming my prayers; many others would attest to something similar.

It is noteworthy that Jesus, in his moment of greatest anguish on the cross, inhabits the words of Psalm 22:1 as his own prayer: "My God, my God, why have you forsaken me?"

In time, the psalms may provide the relevant building blocks for improvisational prayer, as scales and the imitation of other musicians provide the resources for improvisational musicians. But even if this remains difficult, the psalms themselves can be our prayer book. If we never learn to pray improvisationally, we will always have these prayers to read and make our own. If our autistic children continue to struggle with prayer, they can read these prayers for themselves. Parents may need to explain elements of the imagery, of course, which may involve purchasing a good commentary on the psalms. They may also find it helpful to have a concordance to the psalms or to have some other resource that might help them to index the various psalms to particular themes or needs (thanksgiving, repentance, etc.). Learning to use the psalms well, though, may be a vital part of the formational development of persons and families affected by autism, as it should be for every Christian.

There are also books of prayer outside of the Bible that may be helpful for parents to use with their children. Some of these are the great prayer traditions of the church, which might usefully be introduced into the personal piety of those whose tradition (e.g., popular evangelicalism) has come to neglect them. The Book of Common Prayer, for example, may be an invaluable resource to those whose tradition would not normally make use of it. There may also be books prepared specifically for children, or even for autistic children, that could be of benefit; in this age of technology, an app oriented toward meeting the need of autistic individuals for help with prayer could be invaluable. Whatever we do, however, I would suggest that the psalms ought to take a certain priority, to reflect their prominence within the Bible. The danger with substituting other, more contemporary prayers is that these will reflect the deficiencies of our culture of prayer. If the psalms are placed again into the heart of our practices of worship, they have the capacity to model a dramatically more honest and earthy life of faith.

Sexuality

Our next point requires some care, both as we consider the relevant research and as we think about how this might relate to the experience of the person with autism. It will also demand some careful openness to how we read and apply the Bible.

There has been some research in recent years that has suggested a higher correspondence between autism and what we might call "nonstandard sexual identity" than is true of the wider population.[4] The research suggests that autistic people may be more likely to identify with the gender other than their own, or to be homosexual in orientation, or to fit with one of the other categories designated by the acronym LGBTQI. Some may be gender-fluid, identifying differently at different stages of their life. In addition, those whose own sexual orientation or identity is more traditionally aligned with the gender they were assigned at birth may be more open to the legitimacy of nonstandard practices and orientations as others choose to embrace them.

For those whose views on such matters are defined by the more traditional values of their faith, which they consider to be biblical (and exclusively so), this can be troubling. For those with autism, it can create a sense of conflict or mismatch between their own sense of identity and that demanded by their community of faith. For those who are parents or friends of autistic individuals whose sexual identity is incompatible with their own views, it can cause enormous distress, not least because of the conviction that this is a sin that God will punish.

There is no prospect that I can resolve some of the biggest debates going on within the contemporary church in one short section of one short book, and I have no intention of defending any one of the positions that might be taken over against the others. Instead, I will offer some considerations that *ought* to frame the debates and to inform the way they are practiced, but that are generally absent from the discussion. I do so here because the connection with autism means that for some readers this will likely cease to be a debate conducted at a distance, between representatives of different positions, and will instead be a one of immediate pastoral significance or personal relationship, between people with existing relationships that can be fostered or jeopardized by the way we engage in the debate. Some of the relevant points I have already asserted in relation to other issues elsewhere in the book. I will make them again more briefly.

1. Our salvation and our unity are a function of our shared union with Christ, not our agreement on moral or doctrinal matters. This point is glaringly obvious to me in the texts of the New Testament, but is consistently marginalized or even excluded from discussions of Christian unity. In the case of John, it is expressed through various pieces of collective imagery, the strongest of which is the designation of Jesus as the vine and believers as branches (John 15:5). In the case of Peter, it is expressed through the image that "coming to him," the living stone, his people "as living" stones are being built into a spiritual house (1 Pet 2:4-5, my translation). In the case of Paul, it is expressed extensively in the prepositional language of being "in Christ" and the particular imagery that all who have been baptized into Christ have put on Christ, so that "there is no longer Jew or Greek, there is no longer slave or free, there is no longer male and female; for all of you are one in Christ Jesus" (Gal 3:28). For those in the embryonic church described in Acts, this conviction was a difficult one to process, but one that they were forced to by the fact that gentiles were receiving the Spirit in the same way as Jews. Through

Peter's vision in Cornelius' house (Acts 11) and then through their rereading of various Old Testament texts (Acts 15), particularly Amos 9:11-12,[5] they came to recognize that God's act of cleansing had extended beyond the limits that they had expected of it and now included gentiles: "Do not call impure that which God has cleansed" (Acts 11:9, my translation).

This is profoundly important to the discussion about sexuality, because it is often conducted in ways that assume an alternative position is simply incompatible with Christianity and that the person espousing that view is, therefore, not a Christian. As we will note in the next section, this is wrapped up with the question of what is "biblical." We need to remind ourselves that there are examples within the New Testament itself of disagreements over matters of enormous significance, going right down to the very understanding of the gospel, that nevertheless do not compromise the unity of the body of Christ. The disagreement between Paul and Barnabas is often cited as an example of "godly" divergence, but a more important example is that between Paul and Peter (Cephas), which is described in Galatians 2:11, because Peter is quite simply in the wrong, espousing a view that cannot be reconciled with the gospel. Yet Paul does not exclude him from the body of Christ.

That example, in fact, opens a window onto Paul's consistent strategy of moral argument, which is precisely to affirm the fellowship of believers and the unity of the body of Christ as the grounds for moral exhortation. When we read through Galatians, his argument affirms the reality of his readers' experience of the Spirit as the basis for his castigation of their attitude to works. When we read 1 Corinthians, the oneness of the church that is united to the one God through the one mediator, which has been made to drink of the one Spirit, is the basis for his castigation of their manifest disunity in their practices of Eucharist. Applied to this debate, the point is that we make no concession to liberalism when we affirm that those who take a different view than ourselves are equally united to Christ, and we do not minimize the significance of the issue. Quite the opposite: precisely because we are collectively united to Christ, it is more important that the debate happen and that the issues be evaluated carefully, prayerfully, and intensively. But it must be regulated by the principles of love and care that govern the body of Christ.

Now, it is important to recognize that Paul also speaks of a point where someone is to be expelled from the community as an act of discipline. Here, though, we need to recognize two things. First, we can only reach the point of making such a decision when we have considered the issues properly, without foreclosing them on the basis of an a priori assumption that the person at their heart is not a fellow believer. As we have already noted, confronted by the evidence of the spiritual experience of the gentiles, and by Peter's report of his vision, the church in Acts 15 reread their Scriptures, identifying in them meanings and possibilities that they had not previously considered, yet still constrained by the authority of those texts.[6] Second, even the act of expulsion in Paul's scenario assumes that the person is, indeed, a member of the body, for the expulsion is intended to be restorative.

2. The "biblical evidence" is limited and is subject to interpretation; both sides can claim to be "biblical." This statement is probably shocking to many readers, and you may already be marshaling arguments against it, but please read on, at least to the end of the paragraph. To be clear, I am not here saying that the matter is inescapably subjective, or that all readings are equally good. I am saying, instead, that there is only a small amount of material that is relevant to the issue — even if some of it might legitimately be described as of disproportionate significance — and that our reading of this material is governed by a set of interpretive principles that we often take for granted.

The problem here is that the word "biblical" is often thrown around in a very crude way. The passages that directly speak of homosexual activity are relatively scarce, much scarcer than is often assumed. I have in front of me a web page that lists "relevant" biblical texts, labeling these as "Bible Verses about Homosexuality," but the vast majority of them are broadly about sexual immorality or impurity—there is nothing specifically "about" homosexual activity, as the heading claims. In fact, there are only six passages in the Bible that speak of homosexual activity in any direct way (Gen 19; Lev 18:22; Lev 20:13; Rom 1:26-27; 1 Cor 6:9-10; 1 Tim 1:10). The interpretation of these passages is, of course, subject to significant debate: Are they about homosexual activity per se, or about sexual violence (at least in the case of Gen 19)? Does the word used in 1 Corinthians 6:9-10 and 1 Timothy 1:10 (*arsenokoitai*) definitely designate those who practice homosexual acts, or does it refer to some other form of sexual activity, perhaps an exploitative (or exploited) one? Should the labeling of a group as *malakoi* in 1 Corinthians 6:9 necessarily be understood as designating those who practice homosexual acts, when that word simply means "soft ones" and is encountered elsewhere as a description of expensive clothing (Matt 11:8; Luke 7:25, where it contrasts such clothing with the garments of John the Baptist)? To be clear, I do not necessarily consider these challenges to the traditional interpretation to be persuasive, and it is no small task to evaluate them properly, but we need to recognize that they constitute serious and credible challenges to the claim that one particular position can claim, exclusively, to be "biblical."

A case can certainly be made that we should add to this list those texts that seem to present heterosexual marriage as the appropriate "norm" for human sexual expression and that seem to link this to creational order, but here, too, some caution should be exercised. The problem with using creational order as a defining element in Christian ethics is that there are elements of it that appear to be relativized or even redefined in the New Testament. The obvious example is marriage itself, which does not continue into the resurrection state.

> For in the resurrection they neither marry nor are given in marriage, but are like angels in heaven. (Matt 22:30; cf. Mark 12:25)

Luke's account of this story is worded in such a way as to suggest that this principle bears on the current practices of those who will, in future, be resurrected:

> [34] Jesus said to them, "Those who belong to this age marry and are given in marriage; [35] but those who are considered worthy of a place in that age and in the resurrection from the dead neither marry nor are given in marriage." (Luke 20:34-35)

This looks quite similar to what we see in Paul, where singleness is advocated as a desirable, or even preferable, condition for the Christian (1 Cor 7:8-10). For those who see marriage as part of creational order, the affirmation of singleness is a dramatically countercultural move that redefines the normativity of creational order itself. A more subtle, but arguably more significant, example is found in the designation of unclean animals as "what God has cleansed" in Acts 11:9 (my translation). This, of course, is part of the flow of the book of Acts toward its description of the Jerusalem council in chapter 15, where the status of the gentiles is reconsidered. I have mentioned this passage already, as it is an important example (sometimes cited in the debates around sexual identity) of the church reconsidering the teaching of the Old Testament / Hebrew Bible in the light of the gospel and the pouring out of the Spirit. We can easily miss the fact that the cleanness and uncleanness of animals and birds is something linked not to sin but to creational order; things were created "according to their kinds" in Genesis 1 (e.g., 1:21, 24, 25, NIV),[7] and these kinds are categorized as "clean" and "not clean" in Genesis 7:1-10. The words that Peter hears in Acts 11:9 do not indicate that all things were, in fact, created clean, but rather refer to a definitive act of cleansing. The verb form that is used (*ekatharisen*) is aorist: it points to a definitive act by which the status of these creatures has been changed, one that seems to be linked to the sacrifice of Jesus Christ.

These verses do not, of course, indicate that we are in a moral free-for-all, and do not provide support for alternative accounts of sexual identity. But they do prohibit us from seeing the creational order described in Genesis 1–2 as finally normative.

One final point should be noted. Many Christians who remain firmly committed to the normative role of Scripture for Christian thought and life also take seriously the possibility that there are developments or trajectories on moral issues that can be traced back through the Bible but that do not reach their culmination until long after the closure of the canon. Within the Bible itself, these are imperfectly realized, with culturally accepted standards still defining the practices of the church, even as the church constitutes a kind of counterculture, but in time those trajectories are fulfilled. The example of this usually cited is slavery, and it is a very good one: there are no proof texts for antislavery in the Bible, which is one of the reasons that slavery was practiced and perpetrated by Christians for centuries, but there is a coherent account of human dignity and mutual responsibility that eventually led Christians like William Wilberforce to campaign for its abolition. It is an interesting exercise in reflection on such trajectories to read passages like Ephesians 6:5-9, which speak about the relationships between slaves and masters where one or both is a Christian, and then to read the preceding verses about parent/child and husband/wife relationships. We are very comfortable "translating" the passages that affirm slave-master relationships into something more culturally acceptable today, but often reluctant to allow something similar for male-female relationships or sexual identity. Again, my intention here is not to argue in support of a trajectory that affirms a different account of sexual identity, but simply to stress that such an approach does not disregard the normativity of Scripture in the way that it is often seen to do; it is, in fact, no more dismissive of this than most evangelical ethics.

These points collectively highlight that it is less straightforward than we sometimes assume to label one position as "biblical" and another as "unbiblical." We are always making a range of assumptions about what texts say and how they are to be contextualized in relation to other parts of the Bible. For the pastor, parent, or friend of a person with autism whose sexual identity does not conform to traditional expectations, this should bear significantly on how the issue is discussed and evaluated; it should play a significant role in how we seek to "speak the truth in love." The duty of love to other members of the body of Christ obligates us to understand their position, to read their arguments openly and carefully, and, where necessary, to challenge them. Our commitment to Scripture demands that we always be open to the possibility that it might hold us to account for our misreadings of it.

3. We should remember that Christian ethics embrace the whole of life and are oriented toward the flourishing of the believer in Christ. I had originally intended this point to be focused slightly differently, on the need to treat the issue of sexual identity proportionately in relation to other moral issues. I will touch on this point below, but it seems important to frame it in positive terms. The Bible does not shape our lives only through the deployment of commandment—it is a diverse collection of genres that form us in complex ways—but where it does demand certain practices and prohibit others, it does so in ways that are intended to bring about the flourishing of persons and communities, in their mutual relationships to each other and to God, in Jesus Christ. We should not lose sight of this purpose. It is one of the reasons that the commandments and moral principles we encounter in Scripture cover all areas of life, not just those parts of our conduct that are the stuff of taboos.

The problem for us is that we easily lose sight of this and utilize the commandments as means of labeling people as insiders or outsiders of our group. They come to function very easily in relation to our social or symbolic capital, but only when the practices in question are ones that are easily excluded from the group that makes such judgments. So we find it easy to label the person whose sexual identity is different than the one our group upholds as an outsider (often by labeling them in a much more offensive way), and may glibly render this exclusion in very positive ways, as if we are protecting the created order from violations and helping people to flourish sexually. But we find it less easy to deal in such a way with sins like gossip, greed, slander, or laziness; these are commonplace in our churches, and, while we may not endorse them, we also tend not to devote the same energy to denouncing them as we do to certain sexual identities or practices. The Bible does, though. A brief search for the words "slander" and "gossip" shows that the former occurs around thirty times and the latter around ten times. The word "greedy" occurs more than twenty times. I give the figures in general terms because they will vary somewhat between translations, reflecting variation in the underlying Greek and Hebrew. They illustrate, though, the discrepancy between the proportion of space given over by the biblical authors to the challenging of particular attitudes and that given over by us.

I am painfully conscious of how easily this will be misread, so I stress again that I do not write this in order to encourage readers to discard their traditional views, but rather to encourage them to deal in an appropriate way with Christians, including those with autism, whose sexual identity may not conform to traditional norms. Their response should be loving, resistant to the instinct to exclude those who are different and recognizing the bonds of the body of Christ, which are more foundational than moral agreement. It should be humble, recognizing that traditional readings of the Bible may not be fair to its true meaning and may need to be reconsidered. It should still remain faithful, of course, being prepared to hold to unfashionable truths if these remain persuasive. And it should be proportionate, recognizing that the flourishing of Christians and their communities is more widely compromised by things that we are often prepared to accommodate—greed, slander, and gossip—than it is by the things that we readily condemn. We need to reflect on whether our engagement with this issue is distorted by social values.

4. *Each of these points bears on both sides of the argument.* The points just made may be helpful to those who have to deal with a sexual identity—their own or that of another—that does not conform to traditional expectations. They might help us to see that the stark choices we are often forced to make, between remaining in a church that cannot accommodate such differences and leaving the church altogether, may not be necessary. But, at the same time, they demand that those who advocate nontraditional understandings of the biblical texts show love and respect to those who advocate traditional ones. There *is* a biblical case to be made for the traditional understanding of sexual identity and marriage, even if it is possible to critique this and offer an alternative reading of the same material. Furthermore, the obligation to affirm the status of those with whom we disagree as fellow members of the body of Christ, and as fellow readers of Scripture, devolves upon all of us. The command to speak the truth in love constrains every believer, or should.

Autism Reads the Bible

The possibility of distinctively autistic interpretations of the Bible has, to this point, received little attention; what I write here will add little, but will hopefully prompt further study. Do autistic persons read the Bible or practice theology differently, and might their insights be beneficial for others? At first these suggestions may appear problematic. We typically think about "exegesis" as methodologically careful, oriented toward extracting the single meaning of a given passage of Scripture as it reflects the intention of the author; this often goes with an understanding of the task of theology that sees it as an act of assembling exegetical insights into a systematic whole. Conceived in this way, the task of exegesis is essentially "objective," and that of theology builds upon its rigorous findings. The idea that one subcategory of people might read the Bible differently, and/or perform the task of theology differently, would seem to be inadmissible.

This way of conceiving the tasks is problematic, however, as we noted in chapter 2. The task of theology requires us to position the exegesis of any given text within the canonical whole and to relate it to the person of Jesus Christ; this is done, moreover, as an act of "listening" to the word of God, a mode of relationship to the text that is different from that of "analysis." Our theology is our "God-talk," our careful acts of speech that are made in response to this act of listening, which themselves attune us to what we hear and speak to our reading of Scripture. All exegesis is theological, whether we recognize it or not, but the theology that shapes the way we read the text may be good or bad.

Once we recognize this, we can see that those with autism might read the Bible in a way that is particularly constructive and that may be helpful to others. As we noted in chapter 1, those with autism often use language in highly precise ways, something that may allow them to engage with the language play of biblical texts—"the way the words run"[8]—in distinctively careful ways, picking up on features of the text that may be passed over too quickly by a "neurotypical." This, of course, involves some awareness of the place of translation in the functioning of the Bible: the words will always run somewhat differently once they have been translated from one language to another. In addition, the systematizing instinct that often characterizes those with autism might facilitate a distinctive ability to connect texts across the canon, to see correspondences of language or imagery, or to see figural connections. The theological task itself, as an act of careful speech, is one that they may perform with unusual ability, as a result of their instinctively precise and systematic use of language.

If we acknowledge these points, we may speculate on whether some of the great theological exegetes of the past may have been autistic. We cannot allow ourselves to dwell on such speculations, for the same reasons we saw to preclude the diagnosis of biblical characters: we simply do not have access to the relevant data concerning these people. But it is, importantly, quite possible that the church may already have benefited from the abilities of autistic readers and theologians who have not been diagnosed. In addition, as research begins to be devoted to autistic readings of the Bible, one of the factors that may well prove to be important is the presence of as-yet-undiagnosed autism within the community of scholars. There are scholars currently in processes of assessment whose testimonies may cast light on the extent to which autism has already benefited the Christian community.

At present, however, little that has been written on the subject, and few testimonies by autistic people have been offered that might inform it. One interesting example we do have is a short post by Caroline Henthorne, entitled "The Autistic Bible":[9]

It is 1970-something and I am a child in a Sunday school class being told the story of the birth of Moses. It's all rather shocking: the teacher explains that the midwives lied to Pharaoh and that this was the right thing to do! Ten years ago, I was diagnosed as being on the autistic spectrum. Autistic people are by nature honest to the point of bluntness, and suspicious of the idea that it is ever right or necessary to lie. As a child in Sunday school, I had been presented with the all-pervasive cultural assumption of the non-autistics that lies serve some other purpose than obscuring the truth. What if I chose not to believe that?

There has always been debate over how literally to interpret the Bible. It was written, one assumes, in the main, by people who, had they lived today, would not be diagnosed as being on the autistic spectrum. The Bible has its own storytelling style, sometimes poetic in nature, and there are cultural as well as stylistic issues which get lost in translation.

But what if I were to assert my right as a literal thinker, cast in the divine image, to take the Bible at its word and choose to take what the midwives said literally? The results are liberating.

According to Exodus, the Hebrew midwives were told by Pharaoh to kill all the male children at birth. They did not kill them, and they explained to Pharaoh why they hadn't. "The Hebrew women are not like the Egyptian women, for they are vigorous and give birth before the midwife comes to them." I'd like you to consider the possibility that the midwives were brave, not because they dared to lie, but because they dared to tell it like it was: the Hebrew women really did have an easier time giving birth than their Egyptian counterparts. In the west we have assumed that the midwives lied because we could think of no reason why the women of one culture would give birth more easily than those of another. Have we been, like Pharaoh was, wilfully ignorant of women's concerns? I cannot believe that Pharaoh was duped due to ignorance of how children come into the world, or of his culture and its ways.

Henthorne goes on to perceive a correspondence between this story of the Hebrew women, read literally, and accounts of female genital mutilation, as these are rendered in a film by the artist Maryam Tafakory. Henthorne identifies victims of such mutilation as part of the disabled community, dealing with the same complex issues of identity and relationship that she does, as a woman with autism, and needing the same thing that she and the Hebrew women needed: the presence of God.

> My choice to be myself as a disabled woman, and take the Bible literally, has enabled me to see the women disabled through genital mutilation for who they really are: women, who like me, are in need of a God who stands with them. Maryam Tafakory shares, in translation, the name of Moses' big sister, Miriam, who watched over the basket in which the baby Moses was hidden. Before this person represented by Maryam reached the age when I first heard the story of Moses' birth, they had been mutilated in a manner unimaginable to my Sunday school teachers, who I can only assume were unaware that female genital mutilation was practiced in some sectors of Ancient Egyptian society. No one watched over "Maryam."
>
> Centuries after Moses was born, another woman, another of Miriam's namesake in translation, Mary, gave birth. The wonder over the miraculous conception of her child has obscured the ordinary nature of the birth itself. A holy infant was born via a perfectly ordinary vagina. God coming to be with us through an ordinary woman, and no less holy for that. Here is a truth worth telling with all the daring we have.

I am not sure that I agree with this reading of Exodus 1, or grasp all of the connections being made, but the extent to which it illustrates some of the points made earlier in this section is interesting. Henthorne reads the passage in a quite distinctive way and links it, through the figural significance of names (Miriam, Maryam, Mary), to a redemptive understanding of that part of the body that has been mutilated for many women. Her language is bold, avoiding synonyms or euphemisms in the way that is often characteristic of autistic persons, and leads her to a powerful insight about the redemption of the female body. Even if we disagree with the exegetical moves that are made—and such disagreements are the stuff of scholarship, after all—that insight is one that forces fresh theological reflection on an issue that most of us would never discuss.

There may be other, less stark examples of autistic interpretation or theology that benefit the church on a weekly basis through the preaching of pastors with autism. I am aware of at least one such pastor, who is open about his autism and ministers to his congregation in a way that embraces it.[10] I am sure there are countless others of whom I am unaware, and that these numbers will continue to grow as rates of diagnosis begin to catch up with the reality of the life of the church. The serious study of their sermons or teachings could add to our knowledge of how autistic individuals read the Bible in ways that are beneficial for the community as a whole.

As always, though, we need to be careful not to focus on just one part of the spectrum. Others may encounter and process the Bible in ways that remain mysterious to us because they have no capacity for speech or are minimally verbal. We have reflected widely on the distinctive ways in which we might understand God to be at work in the lives of those who are profoundly affected by autism; here I would simply stress the value of allowing our homes and environments to be filled with Scripture, to give as many possibilities as we can for the Bible to be heard or encountered. As we noted earlier in this book, most Christians throughout most of the history of the church have been illiterate and have encountered the Bible through hearing it read by others or through its representation in art. Recovering the place of the spoken word could be invaluable for those with profound autism.

CONCLUSION
Toward a Theology of Autism

In the conclusions to academic monographs, authors usually rehearse and reconsider the main points of their arguments. I will not do so here, but I will make some synthetic observations that draw together a few of the strands that run through the book, highlighting that there are certain common issues that bind the various chapters together, even when they deal with very different issues, and reflecting further upon the significance of these.

A Theology of Weakness and Gift

The theme of "weakness" is a particular characteristic of Paul's theology, though one that, as we saw, draws upon the wider biblical imagery of God's care for the marginal and his delight in choosing them to play a part in his work of salvation. The New Testament, as a canonical whole, opens with a genealogy that emphasizes the place of the marginal and despised in the very gene line of Jesus. When Paul speaks of God's election of the "weak" and "despised" things in 1 Corinthians 1:27-28, he echoes this emphasis as it is reflected more widely in Scripture. The one God works in the same way now that he has always worked in his dealings with humans.[1] When Paul continues to speak of the place of the "weaker" things within the body (1 Cor 12:22), this is an extension of the same point: the things that are naturally or intuitively considered lesser are, in fact, equally important to those that are strong and powerful. They are objects of divine election and love; they are royal gifts to the church; they are functioning members of the body of Christ, without which we would be diminished. Ironically, perhaps, without them the body would be disabled or handicapped. As things that are weak, they may require special care, just as a fragile gift from a royal figure may require cautious handling. The benefits they bring to the body, moreover, may not be obviously linked to their function, in obviously utilitarian terms. They may be impossible to quantify. They are, however, quite real, as those weak things participate in the inexhaustible strength of Jesus Christ, working in and through the parts of his body.

This is an important point, for two reasons. First, as we have seen in chapter 3, it is normal for people to ascribe value to others in the church on the basis of their perceived social capital or strengths. As those who participate in the gospel, we are called to repent of this and embrace a divine perspective on value, through the Spirit's renewal of our mind. "From now on, we regard no one according to the flesh" (2 Cor 5:16, my translation). Second, even when we defend the place of the disabled or the different in society and in the church, we often do so in a way that falls back unwittingly into a kind of utilitarianism. This was illustrated some years ago when the scientist Richard Dawkins indicated in a tweet that he considered it immoral not to abort a baby known to have Down syndrome (a comment for which he later "apologized"); the Down's Syndrome Association responded by writing that persons with Down "can and do live full and rewarding lives, they also make a valuable contribution to our society."[2] As someone who has a relative with Down syndrome, I affirm that point heartily, but we need to be careful not to make the capacity to contribute productively to society the basis for ascribed worth. In the discussion of autism, this is mirrored in the tendency to focus on special abilities or savant qualities when defending the value of persons with autism.[3] While this may be fine for a certain number of people on the autism spectrum, it does nothing to rightly value those who are profoundly affected to the point of being nonverbal, or needing lifelong care. For those who approach the question of value through the gospel, worth is linked to the category of gift, which links it to the giver.

The theology of weakness bears on two further areas. The first concerns the obligation to accommodate the weakness of other parts of the body and to engage with such weakness in loving generosity. As we saw in chapter 4, Paul uses the same language of weakness to speak of those whose qualities of faith do not allow them to enjoy things that are permissible (Rom 14:1–15:4; 1 Cor 8:9-12); those who are strong must not treat this with scorn, but must respond with love, seeking to avoid anything that causes distress to others in the body. While this is not identical to the challenge of accommodating the sensory and social needs of those with autism, it parallels this in useful ways. If we care for those with sensory and social challenges, and see them as part of the body, we will inhabit our freedoms in ways that are caring, forgoing things that are good in themselves, *where appropriate*, in order to accommodate the needs of others.

The second area concerns the struggles of autistic persons with associated problems such as anxiety, depression, and addiction, which we considered in chapter 5. These are manifestations of weakness, where that weakness is understood in terms of one's constitution: the flesh. By recognizing that the gospel is for the weak and that it operates by uniting the weakness of human flesh to the absolute potency of divine strength, we see our weakness recontextualized. It is no longer the last word that defines the possibilities of our lives, but is placed within a bigger sentence that informs its real significance. Within this, the weakness is not simply overridden or left behind, but redeemed and transfigured; God's potency works in and through our weakness, and this participatory quality is vital to the reality of its effects.

Providence, Creation, and New Creation

At various points through this study, we have used the word "providence," though without offering much by way of definition. The study has highlighted the consistency with which God's standards of care for the weak and the marginal are represented as bearing on his involvement with all of creation. He cares for wildflowers that have no utility and unclean birds like ravens, which bring with them the risk of ritual contamination; he chooses the weak and despised things to be members of the body of Christ; he incorporates prostitutes and immigrants into the genealogy of Jesus.

As a doctrine, providence is notoriously fluid and contested, with multiple different definitions through the centuries and across the traditions, some of which are highly problematic.[4] A common feature of the definitions that are generally considered defensible, though, is an emphasis on providence as something that is particular and partitive: it understands God's purpose for *each* creature to be distinctive, rather than simply absorbing everything into a grand scheme for the cosmos. John Webster's definition of the doctrine captures this nicely:

The Christian doctrine of providence concerns God's continuing relation to the world that he has created. In his continuing work of providence, God acts *upon, with and in each particular creature and created reality as a whole*. As God so acts, God preserves created reality and being, maintains its order and directs it to the end that he has established for it. God's providence enacts his enduring love for that which he has made and shows him to be a faithful Creator.[5]

This emphasis is, I think, pastorally significant. God's purpose for each creature is different, even if they share in his purposive involvement in the creation as a whole. His work does not violate the constitution of the creature, even if it is not limited by the natural constraints of that constitution. For those with autism, whether affected in subtle or profound ways, this is an important emphasis. God's purpose (or telos) for each of us is particular, and associated with the particular way that he knitted us together in the womb (Ps 139:13): the one whom he knitted together to be autistic may be led toward a different telos than another person. There are elements of our constitution that are vulnerable to participation in sin and suffering, and these must be transformed by the strength of God, but other elements are particular to our created particularity. The doctrine of providence, with its affirmation of particularity, offers us another strand in our arguments against the tyranny of normality.

This invites us to reflect on what our future state might look like. Will those with autism be healed of their autism in the resurrection? Some will assume that the answer to this is "yes," but actually many of those with autism are troubled by such an idea because their autism is so much a part of their identity, even their redeemed identity.[6]

Certainly, there are passages that suggest the resurrection state to be one that is freed from suffering: Paul's description of the resurrection body as incorruptible and imperishable (1 Cor 15:42-54) would seem to indicate this, and the description of the New Jerusalem in Revelation 22:1-5 describes an end of the curse and the healing of the nations through the leaves of the tree of life. At the same time, the resurrection appearances of Jesus (notably his encounter with Thomas in John 20:26-27) suggest a somatic continuity between the one who is raised and his earthly life; Jesus still bears the wounds of his crucifixion. Arguably, his mortality is transformed and transcended, but it is not obliterated or effaced. This may provide an interesting set of categories for reflecting on how there may be continuity between our current identity as persons with autism and our resurrected condition. To some extent, of course, this is speculative, but it is speculation that exposes a deeper question of whether we genuinely respect and value the one who is autistic by divine providence or whether, deep down, we think they should be otherwise.[7]

On the Community

Throughout this study, I have spoken about believers with autism, and also about the families and caregivers of those with autism. This reflects the fact that we are dealing with a condition that presents in a variety of ways or as a spectrum; many of those with autism are profoundly affected by it and minimally capable of speech, so that it is difficult or impossible for us to comment on whether they should be described as "believers."

It is significant that the Bible tells its stories of God's dealings with communities. There may be particular individuals who are at the focal point of those dealings—Abraham, Sarah, Moses, Deborah, David, Mary, Jesus, Paul, Peter, James, and others—but the dealings are with communities: Israel, Judah, the church. Certain practices generate a solidarity within these communities that is never reducible to the cognitive or spiritual state of one of its members. Circumcision is applied to infants who are days old; Passover is celebrated by those of all ages within a home; other festivals, likewise, create a sense that God is not simply dealing with each person, but with the people as a whole. The lambs are members of the flock, even if only because they continue to be bound to their mother, rather than because they have learned to follow the voice of the Shepherd.

Elements of these symbols are carried forward into the New Testament, where they are modified and newly interpreted in relation to the enacting of faith. Baptism becomes the principal rite of identification with the community that is characterized by faith, and the Lord's Supper takes up the symbolism of Passover and reinterprets it in relation to Christ. Though there are debates within the Christian church about whether baptism should be applied to the children of believers, there remains a strong sense that God's dealings with the individual Christian cannot be separated from his dealings with their community as a whole, including those who are part of that community because of their family connections to it. To repeat: the lambs are part of the flock, regardless of their state of cognitive development.

This allows us to reflect more richly on those examples that we saw of responses to the Spirit of God that cannot be interpreted as a function of cognitive understanding. The unborn John the Baptist leaps in the womb; the Christian who does not know what to pray is assisted by the Spirit to utter groans that cannot be articulated in words. We simply do not know how the Spirit is working in the hearts and neurons of those in our flock who are not yet verbal, who have not reached a point of typical cognitive development and may never do so. They remain part of the flock, however, and our care and hope for them should reflect this.

Leadership

Another of the threads that surfaced at several points in this book has concerned leadership. We naturally value certain characteristics and see them as the stuff of leadership, but, as we saw, that natural or intuitive evaluation may reflect our sinful natures; we want the funny, the smart, and the strong to lead us, but God has chosen the weak things of the world to nullify the strong. Where, then, does this leave the question of leadership?

We have not discussed in this book whether those with autism can be leaders in the church, but it would seem to be the obvious corollary of the points that we have made throughout. It should be obvious, though, that such decisions need to be made wisely, with a realistic and well-informed awareness of the challenges that each person with autism will face in roles of leadership and will bring into the role. Crucially, of course, each person with autism is characterized by different features, and these will bear differently on how each may function within the leadership role. We need to take seriously, for example, that difficulty in understanding nonverbal communication may make it especially challenging for one person with autism to fulfill particular pastoral roles; another person with autism may have no such difficulty. Others may struggle with anxiety and depression, which may not prevent them from acting as pastors and leaders (and may, in fact, enable them to be distinctively insightful in their care), but may require the wider community to be particularly caring of them as the burdens of pastoral encounter weigh upon them. Others may take a refreshingly direct path through the politics of church leadership, but this may itself lead to division if they do not negotiate the social complexities of such situations well. Another may lead a church effectively while privately dealing with the burden of an addiction that they manage, but that is still a dreadful reality for them.

All of this is to say that, in some ways, our willingness to appoint autistic people to positions of leadership may be a test of whether our theology of weakness has really been applied to the church in a thoroughgoing way. If we are willing to affirm them in such roles, our affirmation must be accompanied by a caring support for them in the challenges they face, and perhaps a modification of our perception of the roles that they fill. There are, of course, biblical passages that speak of those roles and of those who should fill them, but ministry and leadership in the present time face all kinds of new challenges, albeit often in ways principally informed by years or decades of cultural traditions.

It is worth noting, in addition, that the particular intellectual skills that some enjoy as a result of undiagnosed autism could well mean that there are many already in pastoral or leadership positions without anyone being aware that they are autistic. They may be thriving, or they may be struggling; in either case, the theology of weakness must govern how their work is valued.

A Final Word on Christian Identity

This book has been intentionally positive about autism. However difficult autism may be for those who are autistic or for their families or caregivers, it must be understood within the category of gift and associated with the goodness of the God who chooses (elects) to involve those with autism in his work and to give them to the membership of the body. Gifts may be fragile and may require to be handled with care; gifts may incur obligations that we might prefer not to have; but they are precious things through which God blesses us in ways that we could never imagine.

While seeking to be positive about autism and to give a rich theological account of it, we also need to be careful not to obscure its *subordinate* significance as a part of our identity. As Christians, our identity is principally defined by our union with Christ. Who we are is principally constituted by who he is: "It is no longer I who live, but it is Christ who lives in me" (Gal 2:20). This is important for those with autism, perhaps now more than ever, because it means that our instinct to embrace that identity must be carefully subordinated to our Christian identity. Christians cannot allow themselves principally to self-identify as "Aspie" or "autistic," terms that are often used to identify the limits of our capacity for change. We can use these labels because they comfort us in the belief that "this is just how I am." Our discussion of the theology of weakness has allowed us to see something important about this: God works in and through our weaknesses, in ways that respect our creaturely particularities, but he really does transform us. What he transforms us into, moreover, is the likeness of Jesus Christ. Each of us may bear that likeness in different ways, but the likeness can be realized in us through the work of the Spirit. Whatever labels we use to describe our identities cannot be given priority over this one: we are in Christ. For in Christ there is no Jew nor Greek, slave nor free, male nor female, able or disabled, autistic or neurotypical, but all are one in Christ.

NOTES

Introduction

1 This term, which is frequently encountered within the autism community as an alternative to "normal people," reflects a concern about the value judgments often associated with our concepts of "normality" and a basic identification of autism as a manifestation of "neurodiversity" rather than disability. We will reflect on the terminology through the course of the book.

2 I began to open this field in a recently published article (Macaskill, 2018a), but this particular book allows me to explore the issues in greater depth than I did there.

3 I am grateful to Sarah Douglas for sharing some insights on this with me shortly prior to the submission of this book.

4 Readers are warmly encouraged to read Brock, 2019.

5 Or as they are known in the UK, "carers."

6 For a helpful review of this show, including this particular scene, see Leslie Felperin, "What Netflix Comedy *Atypical* Gets Right and Wrong about Autism," *Guardian*, 14 August 2017, https://www.theguardian.com/tv-and-radio/2017/aug/14/atypical-netflix-autism-spectrum-depiction-cliches.

7   It should be noted that the preferred convention among healthcare professionals is applied to all conditions, not just autism.

8   Kenney et al., 2016. Quotations taken from abstract.

9   This expression is commonly used in connection with autism advocacy, e.g., as a hashtag item on Twitter.

Chapter 1: Real Autism

1   See the UK National Autistic Society, https://www.autism.org.uk/about/what-is.aspx.

2   In North America, diagnostic practices are informed by the *Diagnostic and Statistical Manual of Mental Disorders* (DSM), which is updated periodically. The current edition is DSM-V (Arlington: American Psychiatric Association, 2013). The rest of the world generally uses the relevant parts of the *International Statistical Classification of Diseases and Related Health Problems* (ICD), also updated on a regular basis. The current edition is ICD 11 (Geneva: World Health Organization, 2018). Both research publications and clinical literature are affected by the differences between these two manuals, and the different timelines for revision mean that North American research can be slightly out of line with that developed elsewhere. The differences are generally minor, but one significant point of divergence concerns the label Asperger's syndrome/disorder, which was removed as a discrete diagnosis from DSM-V, with the broader "autism spectrum disorder" (ASD) preferred and a number of specific forms of ASD itemized. The change is now broadly reflected in ICD 10, but Asperger's syndrome has continued to be used as a diagnosis in the intervening period.

3   See Kanner, 1943, and Asperger, 1944. See the discussion in Silberman, 2015, 88–150. Silberman's work is journalism, rather than research, and there have been some recent developments in views about Hans Asperger (Sheffer, 2018), but it is still a very useful account of the early research and its environments, both political and intellectual.

4   See Freitag, 2007; more recently, De Rubeis and Buxbaum, 2015. A huge number of gene-specific studies are available, indicating that the genetic factors are complex and varied between individuals. The point of note is simply that we have good reason to see autism as connected to gene expression.

5   See the discussion later in this chapter about the claims concerning the MMR vaccination, which have now been thoroughly debunked.

6   This was the original explanation offered by Kanner, 1943.

7   See, for example, Rollins, 2017. This study is focused on one particular gene deletion (16p11.2), but other imaging studies have also noted nontypical anatomical features.

8 This is a live issue in the philosophy of mind. See Piccinini, 2008, who argues that some areas of mind can be considered in computational terms, but not all.

9 The word "expression" here is quite important. We often work with an assumption that our genetic profile straightforwardly determines our development: if we have a particular gene, then we will have a particular physical trait. To some extent, older research into genetics tended to oversimplify how genes were connected to development, even though it recognized that genes were not always "expressed": expression often required certain environmental factors to be present. Someone might be genetically predisposed to certain conditions, such as cancers, but these only occur if certain triggers are encountered. As our knowledge of genetics has progressed, however, and particularly since the completion of the Human Genome Project, we have become aware of the true complexity of how our genes relate to our development, and the issue of expression has become more complicated. One of the factors that has been seen as a possible factor in the genetics of autism is the level of testosterone circulating in the uterine environment. The evidence for this may need to be reconsidered as the gender spread of autism is reevaluated. Until fairly recently, autism was understood to affect males more than females, by a factor of 4 or more. It is now believed to be much more common among females than previously thought, probably being better "camouflaged" by females than in males.

10 See the UK National Autistic Society, https://www.autism.org.uk/about/diagnosis/adults.aspx.

11 Wing, 1981.

12 Asperger, 1944.

13 See Czech, 2018, and Sheffer, 2018.

14 See the entries in both ICD and DSM for this.

15 Silberman, 2015, 64–65.

16 That is, does the word directly signify or label something, or does it function in a way that requires a further level of analogy to make sense? The word "sits" functions differently with respect to literalism in "the dog walks" and in "God walks" (e.g., in Gen 3:8), but grammatically the word has the same precise function. My point is that persons with autism have no trouble with such moves from literal to metaphorical when they observe the precise rules of the language system. By contrast, sarcasm and irony often violate these systems and use language in nonprecise ways, as do some idioms.

17 See Baron-Cohen et al., 2001.

18 See the UK National Autistic Society, https://www.autism.org.uk/about/what-is/pda.aspx.

19 See Bogdashina, 2011 and 2016.

20 The latest definitions offered in ICD and DSM reflect these changes, as does the literature published by, for example, the UK National Health Service.

21 See the discussion above. This is a common label, which is used with neutral significance in the evaluation of autism. Many find it rather distasteful, since it measures levels of functionality against the wider population and implies a judgment on the quality of the person. It is, however, part of the lexicon of autism studies.

22 I use the word "belong" deliberately. We will consider it further in chapter 3, as a word that indicates genuine participation in a community, as distinct from institutional policies of inclusion. As Yong writes, "[Where] the rhetoric of 'inclusion' still suggests that the (ecclesial and institutional) retains some measure of authority in widening the margins, the rhetoric of 'belonging' counteracts such hierarchical and authoritarian tendencies by relocating the power and agency to define the church—the body of Christ and the fellowship of the Spirit—to the people" (Yong, 2016, 262; cf. Swinton, 2012).

23 See Whitehead, 2018. The findings are discussed in a recent article in *Christianity Today*, which considers the exclusion of persons with autism from churches (Briggs, 2018).

24 See chapter 5 for relevant literature.

25 Kanner, 1943.

26 See Silberman, 2015, 47–87, for examples.

27 Stump 2010, 65–81, uses autism to cast light on normal theory of mind and "the second person perspective," by which we enjoy relational knowledge of persons (the "I-You" kind of knowledge), rather than simply factual knowledge (knowledge *that*). Stump's work accepts the theory of mind approach and indicates that those with autism are not capable of a proper knowledge of other persons. This is taken up in, for example, McFall 2016, who applies the term "spiritual autism" to a blindness to God and an inability to relate to his reality. I find it disturbing that the word "autism" can be used in a way that is essentially pejorative. I will return to this point at the end of the chapter, and again in chapter 3. For further criticisms, see also Bustion, 2017.

28 See Baron-Cohen, Leslie, and Frith, 1985. The term "mind-blindness" is widely encountered in the literature, especially from this period.

29 Baron-Cohen, 2011, sees parallels between autism and psychopathy and seeks to differentiate the two on the basis of commitment to moral systems. Much of this is unnecessary, however, if we recognize the essential reductionism involved in identifying empathy directly with its underlying neurophysiological mechanisms.

30 Hamilton, 2013.
31 See Rollins, 2017; Lai et al., 2017.
32 In my view, this is a problem with the account of autism in Stump, 2010.
33 Lai et al., 2016.
34 This may require some reevaluation of one of the areas of research that has been important in the developmental theories, which concerns the circulating testosterone levels in the uterine environment. While the protocols for such studies were good, the findings themselves might reflect some bias of sampling, given that most of the children in question were male.
35 Dunn, Myles, and Orr, 2002; Kern et al., 2006; Bogdashina, 2011 and 2016.
36 Wakefield et al., 1998 (retracted).
37 See Goodlee, Smith, and Marcovitch, 2011.
38 As with Wakefield, 2010.
39 Cox, 2017, 79.
40 Stump, 2010; McFall, 2016.

Chapter 2: Autism and the Bible

1 Bokedal, 2015.
2 Macaskill, 2019; Macaskill, 2018c.
3 Mathew and Pandian, 2010.
4 Mathew and Pandian, 2010, 164 (abstract).
5 "Yahwism" designates the worship of the God whose name is disclosed in the Tetragammaton, YHWH. The name is usually translated as the LORD in the Old Testament, reflecting the reverence with which the name was treated: readers would substitute the word for Lord in the place of the name itself.
6 Torrance, 1969, makes the point in relation to theology that the mode of scientific investigation must be determined by nature of the object of study, a principle that prohibits the simple transfer of scientific methodologies to the study of God. This point can be applied to Scripture, too, although with the important caveat that Scripture participates in the creaturely world of things in history.
7 See the description of these in chapter 1. As a contrastive example of how the biblical material can be read in relation to issues of mental health, see Stuckenbruck, 2013.
8 Novakovic, 2003.
9 See, for example, Ps 51:8.
10 Taylor, 1989; MacIntyre, 1981, 228; Macaskill 2018e, 30–34.
11 See the discussion of the image of God in chapter 3.
12 This is a key principle in Swinton, 2012.

13   The authorship of Colossians is a matter of debate among scholars. For an overview, see Foster, 2016. My own view is that Pauline authorship makes best sense of the presence of Jewish mystical tropes and language in the text. These are discussed by Rowland and Morray-Jones, 2009.

14   Macaskill, 2018d.

15   See Russell, 2004, in toto; Macaskill, 2013, 42–76.

16   Kelsey, 1975 (see also Kelsey, 2009); Vanhoozer, 2002, 125–58.

17   The same observation is made by Hauerwas, 1975.

18   By this, I mean that it is not just the story that is important, but the way the story is told.

19   Macaskill, 2018c, 207–38.

20   The designation of the Bible as a library is widely found through the traditions of the church. It is an important and suggestive image of the diverse modes of biblical authority.

21   Macaskill, 2018c, 207–38.

22   The word "organic" is particularly associated with the Reformed tradition, but what it labels is broadly recognized: the Bible is the word of God, but its composition involves the agency of real, historically located human beings.

23   For this idea, see Malina, 2001, 1–6.

24   Most obviously, the guidance to wives and husbands in Eph 5:21–33. The translation of this passage is not as straightforward as often assumed, since the imperative "submit" is not found in 5:21 in the earliest manuscripts nor in the earliest patristic quotations of the verse. Neither is there a finite form of the verb "submit" applied to wives in verse 24. In both cases, where these early manuscripts are concerned, the language of submission must be carried forward from the participle in verse 20, "submitting to one another." That participle is masculine plural in form, and must therefore be understood to designate the group as a whole.

25   See Olyan, 2008, for discussion of this.

26   See Macaskill, 2018c, in toto, but particularly 207–38.

27   The relationship between Rom 7 and the chapters that flank it, particularly in terms of the assumed identity of the writer, has been the subject of much debate in scholarship. The core question concerns whether Paul writes as a Christian struggling with sin, or whether he here writes from the standpoint of his pre-Christian life. See my discussion in Macaskill, 2019.

28   Properly, he is the Spirit of "his" Son, which takes the identification further into the inner relations of the Trinity.

29   Gorman, 2001.

30   Cf. 2 Cor 4, discussed in chapter 5.

Chapter 3: Autism and the Body of Christ

1   I sketched some of these proposals in Macaskill, 2018a. In this chapter, I will draw upon and develop several of the points made in that article; others will be developed in later chapters.

2   Whitehead, 2018; Briggs, 2018.

3   Much of what I cover in this chapter is paralleled in Yong, 2011, though I actually wrote this chapter before I had read Yong's work. Yong is not specifically concerned with autism (though he does discuss intellectual issues on pages 96–103, in ways that overlap with my own work), but with disability more broadly. His work is warmly commended to the reader who wishes to read more widely on how the Bible can be related to conditions not obviously named within it.

4   The term "Synoptics" labels Matthew, Mark, and Luke, since they share so much material and can hence be looked at together and compared.

5   Evans, 1996.

6   Bauer, 1996, 140.

7   Notably Campbell, 2009.

8   Important studies of the Old Testament / Hebrew Bible in relation to disability include Melcher, Parsons, and Yong, 2017, and Olyan, 2008.

9   See Bauer, 1996. Cf. also Lincoln, 2013, who considers the sexual themes in the stories of the women to be relevant to the perception that Jesus had been conceived outside of marriage. I am less convinced that this theme is important to Matthew, and think that his wider emphasis on the place of the marginal has more explanatory value. The detail of the genealogy is discussed by Bauer, 1996. My discussion here is indebted to his study.

10   This is a notable detail in its own right. In keeping with genealogical practice from the time, Matthew principally names the male line of fathers and sons.

11   Examined in depth by Novakovic, 2003.

12   Freyne, 1998 and 2004; Crossan, 1991. See now the collection of essays in Fiensy and Hawkins, 2013, some of which suggest a range of economic levels were present in Galilee at the time.

13   Several essays in Fiensy and Hawkins, 2013, point to at least some of those in Galilee enjoying a relatively high level of wealth.

14   There is, of course, a backdrop to this. The imagery and language that Jesus uses draw heavily upon those great passages in the Old Testament that speak of God's providential care for his creation (Job 38–41, Isa 40, Ps 104, etc.). When Jesus sets his teaching within this tradition, though, it is particularly oriented toward the ascription of value: God's love attaches itself to the things that the world treats with contempt.

15   The expression is drawn from Crossan, 1991.

16 As does Crossan, 1991. This reflects a tendency to see the Judaism of Jesus' day in wholly negative terms, a tendency that has been widely challenged in recent decades.

17 The Sermon on the Mount, for example, frequently intensifies the moral expectations of the Law.

18 Bockmuehl, 2011.

19 This point is not adequately considered by Burridge, 2007, who prioritizes imitation to an extent that is problematic. Cf. Macaskill, 2019.

20 Cf. Bockmuehl, 1997.

21 See Newman, 1992.

22 One text, 1 Cor 11:7, appears to represent a husband (*anēr*, "a male") *as* the image. This is, though, the exception that rather proves the rule, and it is simply good interpretation to allow the balance of the other texts to control our reading of this one.

23 See, for example, Jewett, 1996, esp. 67. See the discussion in Thomas, 2012. This recognition also lies behind Eiesland, 1994, and the pressure to reconceive the God in whose image we are made as "disabled."

24 I borrow this expression from Kelsey, 2009, where it is used frequently.

25 The language of "dynamic participation," as something linked to, but distinct from, natural participation through the sharing of natures, is developed in Russell, 2004.

26 Russell, 2004. Cf. Macaskill, 2013, 42–76.

27 The best translation of this of which I am aware is Thompson, 1971.

28 *De Incarnatione* 3, trans. Thompson, 1971, 141.

29 While there is not sufficient space to develop the observation here, I would suggest that this participatory way of thinking about the relationship of humans and God is more useful, and theologically defensible, than some of the attempts to present God himself as disabled, as a basis for including disabled persons within the *imago Dei*.

30 Second Corinthians 3:18. The word typically translated "being transformed" is literally "being metamorphosed."

31 NIV and some other versions often simply translate "flesh" as "sinful nature." This is unfortunate, for it masks the fact that the same word is used elsewhere in more neutral terms. See Jewett, 1971, 49–166.

32 Macaskill, 2019.

33 Murphy-O'Connor, 2002.

34 Horrell, 2004.

35 Macaskill, 2018a. My language here is heavily shaped by interaction with the work of Griffiths, 2009. This work concerns the virtuous shaping of intellectual life in general, but his application of the category of "gift" is suggestive and helpful for how we evaluate the cognitive identities of ourselves and others.

36   On the category of "gift" within Paul's theology, see now Barclay, 2015.
37   See Fee, 1994, 427–37. The construction is *hina mē ha ean thelēte tautas poiēte*. The positioning of *ha ean thelēte* before *tautas* suggests that this qualifies what these things are and that the whole construction is subordinated to *hina mē . . . poiēte*. Literally, if awkwardly, "so that not the 'whatever you might wish things' you do."
38   See chapter 1 and chapter 2.

Chapter 4: Autism in the Church

1   Grandin, 2009.
2   LeGoff, 2004; LeGoff and Sherman, 2006; Owens et al., 2008.
3   Swinton, 2012.
4   The construction in Greek actually uses a passive form that indicates the experience of the Spirit to be divinely initiated, rather than a matter of voluntary reception: "we were all made to drink (*epotisthēmen*) of the one Spirit" (1 Cor 12:13).
5   The word used for "participation" is *koinōnia*, which can be translated as "fellowship."
6   Cf. Barclay, 2015.
7   Capitalization mine.
8   See Lai et al., 2016.
9   The Greek verb twice used for "welcome" is *proslambanō*. The verb occurs a number of times in the Greek translations of the Old Testament, closely associated with the idea of God's election of his people. In 1 Sam 12:22, for example, it is used of God's taking to himself a people (this is masked in English translations, since the Hebrew instead has the verb "make"). In Ps 64:5, the verb is used in parallel with the verb "to choose" or "to elect": "Blessed are those whom you elect and welcome to dwell in your courts" (my translation). This links in important ways to the theology of hospitality that some have developed in relation to disability. See Reynolds, 2008.
10   As a welcome example of this, I was recently made aware that the missionary organization Mission to the World (MTW) asks those attending their conferences to avoid wearing scented products.
11   Whitehead, 2018; Briggs, 2018.
12   For comment on "stimming," see chapter 1.
13   Fishbane, 2009.

Chapter 5: The Dark Side of Autism

1   "Comorbidity" is the technical term for the co-occurrence of conditions. I have generally tried to avoid the word in the discussion, as it is one that triggers strong reactions and is subject to misunderstanding by those not familiar with medical terminology.

2   Nah et al., 2018; Croen et al., 2015; Skokauskas and Gallagher, 2010.
3   See Croen et al., 2015.
4   Croen et al., 2015. A useful and accessible treatment is found in Aitken, 2012.
5   Croen et al., 2015, 819.
6   Pandolfi and Magyar, 2016.
7   Pandolfi and Magyar, 2016, 181, referencing Siegel and Beaulieu, 2011.
8   For a powerful personal account of such struggles, reflecting the tension of such difficulties and faith commitments, see Regan, 2014.
9   Croen et al., 2015, suggest lower figures, perhaps through underreporting, or perhaps through failure to diagnose women. See also Butwicka, 2017.
10   See So et al., 2017; cf. Romano et al., 2014.
11   See Cooper, Robison, and Mazei-Robison, 2017.
12   Doidge, 2007; Wilson, 2015.
13   Part of the abstract of Rothwell, 2016, reads:

> One area of overlap involves neural circuits and neuromodulatory systems in the striatum and basal ganglia, which play an established role in addiction and reward but are increasingly implicated in clinical and preclinical studies of ASDs. A second area of overlap relates to molecules like Fragile X mental retardation protein (FMRP) and methyl CpG-binding protein-2 (MECP2), which are best known for their contribution to the pathogenesis of syndromic ASDs, but have recently been shown to regulate behavioral and neurobiological responses to addictive drug exposure. These shared pathways and molecules point to common dimensions of behavioural dysfunction, including the repetition of behavioural patterns and aberrant reward processing.

It is worth noting that Rothwell's article opens with a reference to the lack of comorbidity between autism and addiction. This reflects an older viewpoint (though not significantly older!) that has been challenged by the most recent research.

14   By "exteriority," I mean what the tradition has often labeled as the "alien" reality of righteousness. It originates outside of us, in the person of Jesus Christ, and is never compromised by the limited character of our participation in it. It may, and must, become an interior reality in our lives, but it always originates outside.
15   This verse is not straightforward. It is possible to read the Greek as indicating that names were written before the foundation of the world in the book of the Lamb who was slain. This acknowledges that word order in Greek can be more fluid than in other languages, including English. The expression "from the foundation of the world" (*apo katabolēs kosmou*)

immediately follows the word "slain" (*esphagmenou*, the perfect passive participle of *sphazō*), which is the warrant for understanding the phrase in the way that I have reflected in the main text. The obvious objection to this reading is that Jesus was killed relatively recently (for the author of the book); my point, though, is precisely that the biblical authors see this event as one involving the eternal God, and thus having eternal significance.

16 There are different ways of understanding this. Much scholarship has read this as reflecting the kind of Platonism that is encountered in Philo, the Alexandrian Jewish philosopher roughly contemporary with the New Testament (so Attridge, 1989); others have understood it in terms informed by Jewish apocalyptic or mysticism (so Rowland and Morray-Jones, 2009; Moffitt, 2011; Barnard, 2012).

17 Some traditions have associated the authorship of Hebrews with Paul, but, going back to the early church, this has been a matter of debate. Almost no contemporary scholars, even conservative ones, consider the epistle to be Pauline.

18 See Moffitt, 2011.

19 The term "emergence" has a technical significance, labeling phenomena that are linked to underlying mechanisms or components but cannot be reduced to these, and in themselves are able to affect those underlying elements. The term can be associated with a phenomenon like love, which may emerge from a combination of neural, physiological, and social elements but cannot be reduced to any of these. It is also often linked to the concept of personhood and how this relates to our physical and social constitution: we are more than the sum of our parts, and can never be broken down into these. See Croasmun, 2017.

20 For this, see also Yong, 2011. While I do not disagree with Yong, my own discussion will highlight the connections between physical and moral weakness in a way that he does not.

21 This comparison runs through 2 Cor 3–4. See Heath, 2013.

22 A number of scholars have traced the influence of Paul's Damascus Road experience through his theology. See Kim, 1981; Segal, 1990; and, most thoroughly, Newman, 1992 (revised edition, 2017).

23 Leonard Cohen's song "Anthem" is often quoted in relation to disability, with such connotations:

> Ring the bells that still can ring,
> Forget your perfect offering,
> There is a crack, a crack in everything,
> That's how the light gets in.

24 Classically, the theological traditions have been committed to the concept of divine simplicity, which recognizes that God is one and cannot,

therefore, be divided. Any notion that the oneness of Father and Son breaks down at the cross, or even that the Trinity is broken internally, is theologically problematic, at least in the terms of traditional theology. For an excellent recent treatment of divine simplicity, see Duby, 2015.

25   Fee, 1994, 28–32.

26   Engberg-Pedersen, 2010.

27   My translation is closer to the KJV than to most modern versions, which understand *ektrepō* as "to disjoint" or "to disable"; the verb typically designates some kind of departure from the proper direction of travel, and I would suggest that "fall by the wayside" captures its significance when it is combined with the imagery of lameness.

28   LeGoff, 2004; LeGoff and Sherman, 2006; Owens et al., 2008.

29   I am aware that this is not true of everyone with autism, but for many this will be an attractive and helpful truth.

30   Macaskill, 2019.

31   See, e.g., Snow, 2015.

32   Gabriel and Young, 2011.

33   Cf. Hengel, 1981.

34   Macaskill, 2019.

35   Macaskill, 2018c, 184.

36   This language reflects the classic, Augustinian way of thinking about sin as an inward curving upon ourselves; this is taken up in Luther's theology. See Jenson, 2006.

37   Some with autism may be categorized as having impaired learning, or as having a "mental age" that is different from their biological one. This reflects our standards of what cognitive development should look like at different ages; the point of Matt 11:25 is that it is precisely to those who lack cognitive accomplishment, the infants, that God reveals his great truths.

Chapter 6: Autism and Christian Practices

1   Williams, 2014.

2   This is the basic meaning of *alalētos*.

3   Limb and Braun, 2008; Beaty, 2015.

4   For example, George and Stokes, 2018.

5   See Bauckham, 1995, for an analysis of the use of Amos 9:11-12 according to Jewish reading strategies.

6   Luke Timothy Johnson (2007, drawing on Johnson 1996) has famously argued that the principles and practices of Acts 15, read alongside other important texts, warrant an account of Christian moral reasoning that is able to hold positions that contradict the commandments found within Scripture, particularly on homosexuality. Such new moral positions draw upon experience and the work of the Spirit in this. My own sense is that

the church in Acts 15 continues to consider Scripture normative, and still seeks to read it faithfully according to the principles of Jewish exegesis, but nevertheless reads it in a radically new way in the light of the gentile reception of the Spirit. This is to recognize that the church continues to see itself as constrained by Scripture, but not by its traditional interpretations of Scripture; the key to the new interpretations is that they make sense of new experience using new, but still careful, combinations of scriptural texts. This does not resolve the issue at hand, but gives a different set of categories than those often used, which often focus on the exegesis of specific texts in isolation.

7   The NRSV masks the significance of the underlying Hebrew (*ƚminehem*) and its Greek translation (*kata genos*) by translating as "of every kind."

8   For the relevance of this expression to the use of biblical texts in contemporary psychology and personal formation, see Macaskill, 2018b.

9   See https://www.shapearts.org.uk/blog/the-autistic-Bible. First published in *Reform* magazine, April 2016.

10   Lamar Hardwick is an autistic pastor with an open and strong online presence. See her website at https://autismpastor.com/.

Conclusion

1   Macaskill, 2018e.

2   See https://www.theguardian.com/science/2014/aug/21/richard-dawkins -apologises-downs-syndrome-tweet.

3   The term "savant" designates persons with unusual abilities, sometimes linked to neurological conditions such as autism. The portrayal of autism in the movie *Rain Man* (1988, directed by Barry Levinson, written by Barry Morrow and Ronald Bass) reflected savant syndrome, one of the elements that has caused it to receive criticism for its depiction of the condition.

4   See the essays collected in Murphy and Ziegler, 2009.

5   Webster, 2012, 203 (emphasis added). See also Webster 2009, 158: "Providence is that work of divine love for temporal creatures, whereby God ordains and executes their fulfilment in fellowship with himself. God loves creatures and so himself orders their course to perfection: *mundum per se ipsum regit, quem per se ipsum conditit.*"

6   On the topic of disability in the resurrection, and how this relates to assumed ableist or normate values, see the provocative discussion in Yong, 2011, 118–44.

7   Such issues of identity are at the heart of Yong, 2011.

BIBLIOGRAPHY

Aitken, Kenneth, J. 2012. *Sleep Difficulties and Autism Spectrum Disorders: A Guide for Parents and Professionals.* London: Jessica Kingsley.

Asperger, Hans. 1944. "Die 'Autistischen Psychopathen' im Kinde-salter." *Archiv für Psychiatrie und Nervenkrankheiten* 117: 76–136.

Attridge, Harold W. 1989. *The Epistle to the Hebrews.* Hermeneia. Phila-delphia: Fortress.

Barclay, John. 2015. *Paul and the Gift.* Grand Rapids: Eerdmans.

Barnard, Jody. 2012. *The Mysticism of Hebrews: Exploring the Role of Jew-ish Apocalyptic Mysticism in the Epistle to the Hebrews.* WUNT 2/331. Tübingen: Mohr Siebeck.

Baron-Cohen, Simon. 2002. "The Extreme Male Brain Theory of Autism." *Trends in Cognitive Science* 6: 248–54.

———. 2011. *Zero Degrees of Empathy: A New Theory of Human Cruelty.* London: Penguin.

Baron Cohen, Simon, Alan M. Leslie, and Uta Frith. 1985. "Does the Autistic Child Have a 'Theory of Mind'?" *Cognition* 21: 37–46.

Baron-Cohen, Simon, S. Wheelwright, R. Skinner, J. Martin, and E. Clubley. 2001. "The Autism-Spectrum Quotient (AQ): Evidence from Asperger Syndrome / High Functioning Autism, Males and Females, Scientists and Mathematicians." *Journal of Autism and Developmental Disorders* 31: 5–17.

Bauckham, Richard J. 1995. "James and the Jerusalem Church." In *The Book of Acts in Its First Century Setting*, vol. 4, *The Book of Acts in Its Palestinian Setting*, ed. Richard J. Bauckham, 415–80. Carlisle: Paternoster.

———. 2001. "The Future of Jesus Christ." In *The Cambridge Companion to Jesus*, ed. M. Bockmuehl, 265–80. Cambridge: Cambridge University Press.

Bauer, David R. 1996. "The Literary and Theological Function of the Genealogy in Matthew's Gospel." In *Treasures Old and New: Contributions to Matthean Studies*, ed. David R. Bauer and Mark Allen Powell, 129–59. Society of Biblical Literature Symposium Series 1. Atlanta: Scholars Press.

Beaty, R. E. 2015. "The Neuroscience of Musical Improvisation." *Neuroscience and Biobehavioural Reviews* 51: 108–17.

Bitner, Bradley. 2015. *Paul's Political Strategy in 1 Corinthians 1–4: Constitution and Covenant.* SNTS Monograph Series 163. Cambridge: Cambridge University Press.

Blakemore, S.-J., T. Tavassoli, S. Calò, R. M. Thomas, C. Catmur, U. Frith, and P. Haggard. 2006. "Tactile Sensitivity in Asperger Syndrome." *Brain and Cognition* 61: 5–13.

Bockmuehl, Markus. 1997. "The Form of God (Phil 2:6): Variations on a Theme of Jewish Mysticism." *Journal of Theological Studies* 48: 1–23.

———. 2011. "The Trouble with the Inclusive Jesus." *Horizons in Biblical Theology* 33: 9–23.

Bogdashina, Olga. 2011. *Autism and the Edges of the Known World: Sensitivities, Language and Constructed Reality.* London: Jessica Kingsley.

Bogdashina, Olga. 2016. *Sensory Perceptual Issues in Autism and Asperger Syndrome: Different Sensory Experiences, Different Sensory Worlds.* 2nd ed. London: Jessica Kingsley.

Bokedal, Tomas. 2015. "The Early Rule-of-Faith Pattern as Emergent Biblical Theology." *Theofilos* 7 (1) (suppl.): 57–75.

Briggs, David. 2018. "Study: US Churches Exclude Children with Autism, ADD/ADHD." *Christianity Today.* July 20. https://www.christianitytoday.com/ct/2018/july-web-only/study-us-churches-exclude-children-with-autism-addadhd.html.

Briggs, Richard. 2010. *The Virtuous Reader: Old Testament Narrative and Interpretive Virtue*. Grand Rapids: Baker.

Brock, Brian. 2019. *Wondrously Wounded: Theology, Disability, and the Body of Christ*. Waco: Baylor University Press.

Brown, William P., ed. 2003. *Character and Scripture: Moral Formation, Community, and Biblical Interpretation*. Grand Rapids: Eerdmans.

Burridge, Richard. 2007. *Imitating Jesus: An Inclusive Approach to New Testament Ethics*. Grand Rapids: Eerdmans.

Bustion, Olivia. 2017. "Autism and Christianity: An Ethnographic Intervention." *Journal of the American Academy of Religion* 85: 653–81.

Butwicka, Agnieszka. 2017. "Increased Risk for Substance Use-Related Problems in Autism Spectrum Disorders: A Population-Based Cohort Study." *Journal of Autism and Developmental Disorders* 47: 80–89.

Campbell, Douglas. 2009. *The Deliverance of God: An Apocalyptic Re-reading of Justification in Paul*. Grand Rapids: Eerdmans.

Christensen, Deborah L., Jon Baio, Kim Van Naarden Braun, Deborah Bilder, Jane Charles, John N. Constantino, Julie Daniels, et al. 2016. "Prevalence and Characteristics of Autism Spectrum Disorder among Children Aged 8 Years—Autism and Developmental Disabilities Monitoring Network, 11 Sites, United States, 2012." Morbidity and Mortality Weekly Report. *Surveillance Summaries* 65: 1–23.

Cooper S., A. J. Robison, and M. S. Mazei-Robison. 2017. "Reward Circuitry in Addiction." *Neurotherapeutics* 14: 687–97.

Cox, Jennifer Anne. 2017. *Autism, Humanity and Personhood: A Christ-Centred Theological Anthropology*. Newcastle upon Tyne: Cambridge Scholars.

Craig, M. C., S. H. Zaman, E. M. Daly, W. J. Cutter, D. M. Robertson, B. Hallahan, F. Toal, et al. 2007. "Women with Autistic-Spectrum Disorder: Magnetic Resonance Imaging Study of Brain Anatomy." *British Journal of Psychiatry* 191: 224–28.

Crane, Laura, Lorna Goddard, and Linda Pring. 2013. "Sensory Processing in Adults with Autism Spectrum Disorders." *Autism* 13: 215–28.

Croasmun, Matthew. 2017. *The Emergence of Sin: The Cosmic Tyrant in Romans*. Oxford: Oxford University Press.

Croen, Lisa A., Ousseny Zerbo, Yinge Qian, Maria L. Massolo, Steve Rich, Stephen Sidney, and Clarissa Kripke. 2015. "The Health Status of Adults on the Autism Spectrum." *Autism* 19: 814–23.

Crossan, John Dominic. 1991. *The Historical Jesus: The Life of a Jewish Galilean Peasant.* Edinburgh: T&T Clark. Repr., New York: Harper and Row, 1993.

Czech, Herwig. 2018. "Hans Asperger, National Socialism, and 'Race Hygiene' in Nazi-Era Vienna." *Molecular Autism* 9: 29.

De Rubeis, S., and J. D. Buxbaum. 2015. "Genetics and Genomics of Autism Spectrum Disorder: Embracing Complexity." *Human Molecular Genetics* 24: 24–31.

Doidge, Norman. 2007. *The Brain That Changes Itself: Stories of Personal Triumph from the Frontiers of Brain Science.* London: Penguin.

Duby, Steven. 2015. *Divine Simplicity: A Dogmatic Account.* London: T&T Clark.

Dunn, W., B. S. Myles, and S. Orr. 2002. "Sensory Processing Issues Associated with Asperger Syndrome: A Preliminary Investigation." *American Journal of Occupational Therapy* 56: 97–102.

Eiesland, Nancy. 1994. *The Disabled God: Toward a Liberatory Theology of Disability.* Nashville: Abingdon.

Engberg-Pedersen, Troels. 2010. *Cosmology and Self in the Apostle Paul: The Material Spirit.* Oxford: Oxford University Press.

Evans, C. Stephen. 1996. *The Historical Christ and the Jesus of Faith.* Oxford: Oxford University Press.

Fee, Gordon. 1994. *God's Empowering Presence: The Holy Spirit in the Letters of Paul.* Peabody: Hendrickson.

Fiensy, David A., and Ralph K. Hawkins, eds. 2013. *The Galilean Economy in the Time of Jesus.* Early Christianity and Its Literature 11. Atlanta: Society of Biblical Literature Press.

Fishbane, Michael. 2009. *Sacred Attunement: A Jewish Theology.* Chicago: University of Chicago Press.

Foster, Paul. 2016. *Colossians.* Black's New Testament Commentaries. London: Bloomsbury.

Freitag, C. M. 2007. "The Genetics of Autistic Disorders and Its Clinical Relevance: A Review of the Literature." *Molecular Psychiatry* 12: 2–22.

Freyne, Seán. 1998. *Galilee: From Alexander the Great to Hadrian, 323 BCE–135 CE.* 2nd ed. Edinburgh: T&T Clark.

———. 2004. *Jesus, a Jewish Galilean: A New Reading of the Jesus Story.* London: T&T Clark Continuum.

Gabriel, Shira, and Ariana F. Young. 2011. "Becoming a Vampire without Being Bitten: The Narrative Collective-Assimilation Hypothesis." *Psychological Science* 22: 990–94.

George R., and M. A. Stokes. 2018. "Sexual Orientation in Autism Spectrum Disorder." *Autism Research* 11: 133–41.

Goodlee, Fiona, Jane Smith, and Harvey Marcovitch. 2011. "Editorial: Wakefield's Article Linking MMR Vaccine and Autism Was Fraudulent." *British Medical Journal* 342.

Gorman, Michael. 2001. *Cruciformity: Paul's Narrative Spirituality of the Cross*. Grand Rapids: Eerdmans.

Grandin, Temple. 2009. "How Does Visual Thinking Work in the Mind of a Person with Autism? A Personal Account." *Philosophical Transactions B* 364 (1522): 1437–42.

Grandin, Temple, and Richard Panek. 2013. *The Autistic Brain: Helping Different Kinds of Minds Succeed*. New York: Mariner Books.

Grandin, Temple, and Margaret M. Scariano. 1986. *Emergence–Labeled Autistic*. Novato: Arena Press.

Griffiths, Paul. 2009. *Intellectual Appetite: A Theological Grammar*. Washington, D.C.: Catholic University of America Press.

Hamilton, Antonia F. de C. 2013. "Reflecting on the Mirror Neuron System in Autism: A Systematic Review of Current Theories." *Developmental Cognitive Neuroscience* 3: 91–105.

Hauerwas, Stanley. 1975. *Character and Christian Life: A Study in Theological Ethics*. San Antonio: Trinity University Press.

Heath, Jane. 2013. *Paul's Visual Piety: The Metamorphosis of the Believer*. Oxford: Oxford University Press.

Hengel, Martin. 1981. *The Atonement: The Origins of the Doctrine in the New Testament*. London: SCM Press.

Holland, Glen. 2016. "'Delivery, Delivery, Delivery': Accounting for Performance in the Rhetoric of Paul's Letters." In *Paul and Ancient Rhetoric: Theory and Practice in the Hellenistic Context*, ed. Stanley Porter and Bryan Dyer, 119–40. Cambridge: Cambridge University Press.

Horrell, David. 2004. "Domestic Space and Christian Meetings at Corinth: Imagining New Contexts and the Buildings East of the Theatre." *New Testament Studies* 50: 349–69.

James, William H. 2014. "An Update on the Hypothesis That One Cause of Autism Is High Intrauterine Levels of Testosterone of Maternal Origin." *Journal of Theoretical Biology* 355: 33–39.

Jenson, Matt. 2006. *The Gravity of Sin: Augustine, Luther and Barth on "homo incurvatus in se."* London: T&T Clark.

Jewett, Paul K., with Marguerite Schuster. 1996. *Who We Are: Our Dignity as Human; A Neo-Evangelical Theology*. Grand Rapids: Eerdmans.

Jewett, Robert. 1971. *Paul's Anthropological Terms: A Study of Their Use in Conflict Setttings*. Leiden: Brill.

Johnson, Luke Timothy. 1996. *Scripture and Discernment: Decision-Making in the Church*. Nashville: Abingdon.

———. 2007. "Homosexuality and the Church: Scripture and Experience." *Commonweal Magazine*, June 11, 2007, 1–5. https://www.commonwealmagazine.org/homosexuality-church-0.

Kanner, Leo. 1943. "Autistic Disturbances of Affective Contact." *Nervous Child* 2: 217–50.

Kelsey, David. 1975. *The Uses of Scripture in Recent Theology*. London: SCM Press.

———. 2009. *Eccentric Existence: A Theological Anthropology*. 2 vols. Louisville: Westminster John Knox.

Kenney, Lorcan, Caroline Hattersley, Bonnie Molins, Carole Buckley, Carol Povey, and Elizabeth Pellicano. 2016. "Which Terms Should Be Used to Describe Autism? Perspectives from the UK Autism Community." *Autism* 20: 442–62.

Kern, J. K., M. H. Trivedi, C. R. Garver, B. D. Grannemann, A. A. Andrews, J. S. Savla, D. G. Johnson, et al. 2006. "The Pattern of Sensory Processing Abnormalities in Autism." *Autism* 10: 480–94.

Kim, Seyoon. 1981. *The Origin of Paul's Gospel*. WUNT 2/4. Tübingen: Mohr Siebeck.

Kim, Young Shin, Bennett L. Leventhal, Yun-Joo Koh, Eric Fombonne, Eugene Laska, Eun-Chung Lim, Keun-Ah Cheon, et al. 2011. "Prevalence of Autism Spectrum Disorders in a Total Population." *American Journal of Psychiatry* 168: 904–12.

Lai, Meng-Chuan, Jason P. Lerch, Dorothea L. Floris, Amber N. V. Ruigrok, Alexa Pohl, Michael V. Lombardo, and Simon Baron-Cohen. 2017. "Imaging Sex/Gender and Autism in the Brain: Etiological Implications." *Journal of Neuroscience Research* 95: 380–97.

Lai, Meng-Chuan, Michael V. Lombardo, Amber N. V. Ruigrok, Bhismadev Chakrabarti, Bonnie Auyeung, Peter Szatmari, Francesca Happé, and Simon Baron-Cohen. 2016. "Quantifying and Exploring Camouflaging in Men and Women with Autism." *Autism* 21: 690–702.

Lawrence, Louise. 2013. *Sense and Stigma in the Gospels: Depictions of Sensory-Disabled Characters*. Oxford: Oxford University Press.

LeGoff, D. 2004. "Use of LEGO® as a Therapeutic Medium for Improving Social Competence." *Journal of Autism and Developmental Disorders* 34: 557–71.

LeGoff, D., and M. Sherman. 2006. "Long-Term Outcome of Social Skills Intervention Based on Interactive LEGO® Play." *Autism* 10: 317–29.

Limb, C. J., and A. R. Braun. 2008. "Neural Substrates of Spontaneous Musical Performance: An FMRI Study of Jazz Improvisation." *PLOS One.*

Lincoln, Andrew. 2013. *Born of a Virgin: Reconceiving Jesus in the Bible, Tradition and Theology.* London: SPCK.

Macaskill, Grant. 2007. *Revealed Wisdom and Inaugurated Eschatology in Ancient Judaism and Early Christianity.* Supp. Journal for the Study of Judaism 115. Leiden: Brill.

———. 2013. *Union with Christ in the New Testament.* Oxford: Oxford University Press.

———. 2018a. "Autism Spectrum Disorders and the New Testament: Preliminary Reflections." *Journal of Disability and Religion* 22: 15–41.

———. 2018b. "Christian Scriptures and the Formation of Intellectual Humility." *Journal of Psychology and Theology* 46: 243–52.

———. 2018c. *The New Testament and Intellectual Humility.* Oxford: Oxford University Press.

———. 2018d. "Union(s) with Christ: Colossians 1:15–20." *Ex Auditu* 33: 92–107.

———. 2018e. "The Way the One God Works: Covenant and Ethics in 1 Corinthians." In *One God, One People, One Future: Essays in Honour of N. T. Wright,* ed. John Dunne and Eric Llewellyn, 112–25. London: SPCK.

———. 2019. *Living in Union with Christ: Paul's Gospel and Christian Moral Identity.* Grand Rapids: Baker Academic.

MacIntyre, Alasdair. 1981. *After Virtue: A Study in Moral Theory.* Notre Dame: University of Notre Dame Press.

Malina, Bruce. 2001. *The New Testament World: Insights from Cultural Anthropology.* Louisville: John Knox.

Martyn, J. Louis. 1997. *Galatians: A New Translation with Introduction and Commentary.* Anchor Yale Bible 33. New York: Doubleday. Repr., New Haven: Yale University Press, 2010.

Mathew, Stephen K., and Jeyaraj D. Pandian. 2010. "Newer Insights to the Neurological Diseases among Biblical Characters of Old Testament." *Annals of Indian Academy of Neurology* 13: 164–66.

McFall, Michael T. 2016. "Divine Hiddenness and Spiritual Autism." *Heythrop Journal* 57 (6). Published online.

Melcher, Sarah J., Mikeal C. Parsons, and Amos Yong, eds. 2017. *The Bible and Disability: A Commentary.* Waco: Baylor University Press.

Moffitt, David. 2011. *Atonement and the Logic of the Resurrection in Hebrews.* Supp. Novum Testamentum 141. Leiden: Brill.

Murphy, Francesca Aran, and Philip G. Ziegler, eds. 2009. *The Providence of God.* London: T&T Clark.

Murphy-O'Connor, Jerome. 2002. *St. Paul's Corinth: Text and Archaeology.* Rev. ed. Collegeville, Minn.: Liturgical Press.

Nah, Y. H., N. Brewer, R. L. Young, and R. Flower. 2018. "Brief Report: Screening Adults with Autism Spectrum Disorder for Anxiety and Depression." *Journal of Autism and Developmental Disorders* 48: 1841–46.

Newman, Carey C. 1992. *Paul's Glory-Christology: Tradition and Rhetoric.* Leiden: Brill. Repr., Waco: Baylor University Press, 2017.

Novakovic, Lidija. 2003. *Messiah, the Healer of the Sick: A Study of Jesus as the Son of David in the Gospel of Matthew.* WUNT 2/170. Tübingen: Mohr Siebeck.

Olyan, Saul M. 2008. *Disability in the Hebrew Bible: Interpreting Mental and Physical Differences.* Cambridge: Cambridge University Press.

Owens, G., Y. Granader, A. Humphrey, and S. Baron-Cohen. 2008. "LEGO® Therapy and the Social Use of Language Programme: An Evaluation of Two Social Skills Interventions for Children with High Functioning Autism and Asperger Syndrome." *Journal of Autism and Developmental Disorders* 38: 1944–57.

Pandolfi, Vincent, and Caroline I. Magyar. 2016. "Psychopathologies." In *Comorbid Conditions among Children with Autism Spectrum Disorders,* ed. Johnny Matson, 171–86. Autism and Child Psychology Series 10. Cham: Springer.

Piccinini, Gualtiero. 2008. "Some Neural Networks Compute, Others Don't." *Neural Networks* 21: 311–21.

Planche, Pascal, and Eric Lemmonier. 2012. "Children with High-Functioning Autism and Asperger's Syndrome: Can We Differentiate Their Cognitive Profiles?" *Research in Autism Spectrum Disorders* 6: 939–48.

Porter, Stanley, and Bryan Dyer, eds. 2016. *Paul and Ancient Rhetoric: Theory and Practice in the Hellenistic Context.* Cambridge: Cambridge University Press.

Regan, Tessie. 2014. *Shorts: Stories about Alcohol, Asperger Syndrome and God.* London: Jessica Kingsley.

Reynolds, Thomas E. 2008. *Vulnerable Communion: A Theology of Disability and Hospitality.* Grand Rapids: Brazos.

Rollins, Nancy. 2017. "An Imaging Glimpse into the Autistic Brain." *Radiology* 286: 227–28.

Romano, Michela, Roberto Truzoli, Lisa A. Osborne, and Phil Reed. 2014. "The Relationship between Autism Quotient, Anxiety, and Internet Addiction." *Research in Autism Spectrum Disorders* 8: 1521–26.

Rothwell, Patrick E. 2016. "Autism Spectrum Disorders and Drug Addiction: Common Pathways, Common Molecules, Distinct Disorders?" *Frontiers in Neuroscience.* February.

Rowland, Christopher, and Christopher Morray-Jones. 2009. *The Mystery of God: Early Jewish Mysticism and the New Testament.* Compendia rerum Iudaicarum ad Novum Testamentum 3:12. Leiden: Brill.

Russell, Norman. 2004. *The Doctrine of Deification in the Greek Patristic Tradition.* Oxford: Oxford University Press.

Segal, Alan. 1990. *Paul the Convert: The Apostolate and Apostasy of Saul the Pharisee.* New Haven: Yale University Press.

Sheffer, Edith. 2018. *Asperger's Children: The Origins of Autism in Nazi Vienna.* London: W. W. Norton.

Siegel, M., and A. Beaulieu. 2011. "Psychotropic Medications in Children with Autism Spectrum Disorders: A Systematic Review and Synthesis for Evidence-Based Practice." *Journal of Autism and Developmental Disorders* 42: 1592–1605.

Silberman, Steve. 2015. *NeuroTribes: The Legacy of Autism and the Future of Neurodiversity.* New York: Avery.

Skokauskas, N., and L. Gallagher. 2010. "Psychosis, Affective Disorders and Anxiety in Autistic Spectrum Disorder: Prevalence and Nosological Considerations." *Psychopathology* 43: 8–16.

Snow, Nancy E., ed. 2015. *Cultivating Virtue: Perspectives from Philosophy, Theology, and Psychology.* Oxford: Oxford University Press.

So, Ryuhei, Kazunori Makino, Masaki Fujiwara, Tomoya Hirota, Kozo Ohcho, Shin Ikeda, Shouko Tsubouchi, and Masatoshi Inagaki. 2017. "The Prevalence of Internet Addiction among a Japanese Adolescent Psychiatric Clinic Sample with Autism Spectrum Disorder and/or Attention-Deficit Hyperactivity Disorder: A Cross-Sectional Study." *Journal of Autism and Developmental Disorders* 47: 2217–24.

Stuckenbruck, Loren. 2013. "The Human Being and Demonic Invasion: Therapeutic Models in Ancient Jewish and Christian Texts." In *Spirituality, Theology, and Mental Health: Multidisciplinary Perspectives*, ed. Christopher C. H. Cook, 94–119. London: SCM Press.

Stump, Eleonore. 2010. *Wandering in Darkness: Narrative and the Problem of Suffering*. Oxford: Oxford University Press.

Swinton, John. 2012. "From Inclusion to Belonging: A Practical Theology of Community, Disability and Humanness." *Journal of Religion, Disability and Health* 16: 172–90.

Tanner, Kathryn. 2001. *Jesus, Humanity and the Trinity: A Brief Systematic Theology*. Edinburgh: T&T Clark.

———. *Christ the Key*. Cambridge: Cambridge University Press.

Taylor, Charles. 1989. *The Sources of the Self: The Making of Modern Identity*. Cambridge, Mass.: Harvard University Press.

Thomas, Philip. 2012. "The Relational-Revelational Image: A Reflection on the Image of God in the Light of Disability and on Disability in the Light of the Image of God." *Journal of Disability and Religion* 16: 133–53.

Thompson, Robert, ed. and trans. 1971. *Athanasius: Contra Gentes and De Incarnatione*. Oxford: Clarendon.

Torrance, Thomas F. 1969. *Theological Science*. Oxford: Oxford University Press.

Vanhoozer, Kevin. 2002. *First Theology*. Leicester: Apollos.

Wakefield, Andrew J., et al. 1998 (retracted). "Ileal-lymphoid-nodular Hyperplasia, Non-specific Colitis, and Pervasive Developmental Disorder in Children." *Lancet* 351: 637–41.

Wakefield, Andrew J. 2010. *Callous Disregard: Autism and Vaccines; The Truth behind a Tragedy*. New York: Skyhorse.

Webster, John B. 2009. "On the Theology of Providence." In *The Providence of God*, ed. Francesca Aran Murphy and Philip G. Ziegler, 158–77. London: T&T Clark.

———. 2012. "Providence." In *Mapping Modern Theology: A Thematic and Historical Introduction*, ed. Kelly M. Kapic and Bruce L. McCormack, 203–26. Grand Rapids: Baker.

Whitehead, Andrew L. 2018. "Religion and Disability: Variation in Religious Service Attendance Rates for Children with Chronic Health Conditions." *Journal for the Scientific Study of Religion* 57: 377–95.

Williams, Rowan. 2014. *The Edge of Words: God and the Habits of Language*. London: Bloomsbury.

Wilson, Gary. 2015. *Your Brain on Porn: Internet Pornography and the Emerging Science of Addiction*. Margate: Commonwealth.

Wing, Lorna. 1981."Asperger's Syndrome: A Clinical Account." *Psychological Medicine* 11: 115–29.

Yong, Amos. 2011. *The Bible, Disability, and the Church: A New Vision of the People of God*. Grand Rapids: Eerdmans.

————. 2016. "Disability and the Renewal of Theological Education: Beyond Ableism." In *Theology and the Experience of Disability: Interdisciplinary Perspectives from Voices Down Under*, ed. Andrew Picard and Myk Habets, 250–62. London: Routledge.

AUTHOR INDEX

SCRIPTURE INDEX

SUBJECT INDEX